PET Scan in Hodgkin Lymphoma

Andrea Gallamini

Editor

PET Scan in Hodgkin Lymphoma

Role in Diagnosis, Prognosis, and Treatment

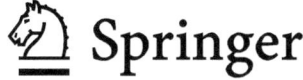 Springer

Editor
Andrea Gallamini
Research, Innovation and Statistics
A. Lacassagne Cancer Center
Nice
France

ISBN 978-3-319-31795-3   ISBN 978-3-319-31797-7   (eBook)
DOI 10.1007/978-3-319-31797-7

Library of Congress Control Number: 2016944145

Printed on acid-free paper

This Springer imprint is published by Springer Nature
The registered company is Springer International Publishing AG Switzerland

Contents

Martin Hutchings, Annika Loft, and Tarec Christoffer El-Galaly

1.1 Historical Background

Accurate baseline staging of Hodgkin lymphoma (HL) is crucial for prognostication and guides important treatment decisions. This remains true in the era of highly effective combined modality treatments and intensive multi-agent chemotherapy regimens that lead to cure in the vast majority of HL patients irrespective of disease stage [1, 2]. In the early 1970s the Committee on Hodgkin's Disease Staging Classification convened in Ann Arbor, Michigan, and this resulted in the first staging classification for HL which was named after the city [3]. The Ann Arbor staging classification became the widely accepted classification for disease staging in HL and enabled comparison of studies by different investigators. The main clinical purpose of the Ann Arbor Classification was to accurately identify patients with limited-stage HL who could be treated with a curative intent with radiotherapy alone. Accurate staging was pursued through rigorous procedures, which included both a clinical and a pathological staging workup. Clinical stage was determined from physical examination, symptom assessment, lymphangiograms, and radiograms, some of which are still elements in modern HL staging. Pathological stage was derived from the results of invasive staging procedures including diagnostic laparotomy and iliac crest bone marrow biopsy (BMB). The risk of serious complications and discomfort related to invasive procedures were tolerated at that time as no good alternatives for evaluation of deep lymph node regions and organs were available. The introduction of computed tomography (CT) enabled noninvasive assessment of deep lymph node regions/organs and changed the staging of HL fundamentally. The committee convened to discuss the evaluation and staging of patients with Hodgkin's disease met in the Cotswolds (UK) and the report generated by the committee recommended CT of the thorax and abdomen in the routine staging workup of HL. Invasive staging procedures with the exception of iliac crest bone marrow biopsy were no longer considered necessary (Cotswold modifications of the Ann Arbor Classification) [4].

M. Hutchings (✉)
Department of Haematology, Rigshospitalet,
Blegdamsvej 9, DK-2100 Copenhagen, Denmark
e-mail: martin.hutchings@gmail.com

A. Loft
Department of Clinical Physiology and Nuclear
Medicine – PET and Cyclotron Unit, Rigshospitalet,
Blegdamsvej 9, DK-2100 Copenhagen, Denmark
e-mail: annika.loft.jakobsen@regionh.dk

T.C. El-Galaly
Department of Hematology, Aalborg University
Hospital, Moelleparkvej 4, DK-9100 Aalborg,
Denmark
e-mail: tarec.galaly@gmail.com

1.2   The Introduction of Functional Imaging

The introduction of functional imaging was another shift in paradigm and defined the current era of modern HL staging. From a CT-based disease staging relying on the size of lymph nodes and morphological abnormalities in organs, functional imaging now provides information on local metabolic activity. This is a major advantage, since knowledge of local metabolism can facilitate discrimination between active HL and nonmalignant morphological abnormalities as well as visualize HL lesions in areas without clear morphological abnormalities. The first functional imaging method to enhance the accuracy of HL staging was the whole-body ^{67}gallium scintigraphy, but this procedure is laborious and the image quality often rather poor. After the introduction of positron emission tomography (PET), gallium scans quickly disappeared from

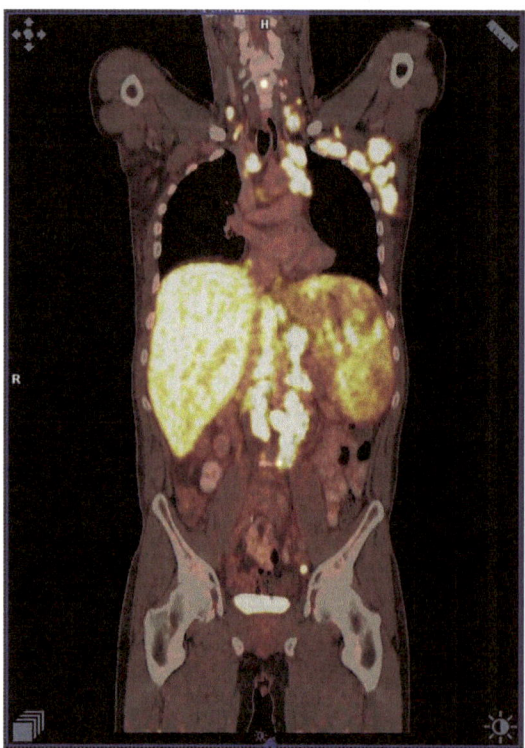

Fig. 1.1 Fusion PET/CT image of a patient with stage IV HL, showing disease in lymph nodes above and below the diaphragm, as well as in the spleen and liver

the management of HL. The most common PET tracer is the radioactive glucose analogue ^{18}F-flurodeoxyglucose (FDG). This tracer is widely studied in HL and FDG-PET is the only type of functional imaging that has been implemented in the routine management of the disease. FDG-PET (in the following referred to as PET) provides a whole-body map of glucose metabolism and HL lesions were found to be universally PET positive (except for very small lesions below the spatial resolution of PET) [5]. An important limitation of stand-alone PET is the inability to locate the exact anatomical area of increased glucose metabolism. This was overcome with the introduction of integrated PET/CT scanner, which made it possible to perform both PET and CT in a single procedure, using CT for attenuation correction of PET data, and to demonstrate the anatomical localization of areas with increased glucose metabolism seen on PET. In this way, modern imaging enables clinically relevant functional and anatomical information to be obtained together. CT and PET can be viewed separately, side-by-side and "fused" with the PET scan overlaid on the CT in color. Today, PET studies are almost exclusively performed with integrated PET/CT machines (Fig. 1.1).

1.3   Early Studies of Staging PET

PET is more sensitive and specific than CT because abnormal FDG uptake may be observed in normal-sized nodes and also seen without changes in organ architecture, e.g., in the liver, spleen, and bones. Over the past 20 years, a number of studies have demonstrated the increased sensitivity of PET relative to conventional imaging.

In their study published in 1998, Bangerter et al. scanned 44 HL patients as a part of their initial staging workup. PET and conventional staging were concordant in 128 (96 %) of 133 diseased lymph node regions. Six patients changed stage as a result of PET, five being upstaged and one downstaged, leading to a change of treatment strategy in all six patients.

This study was the first to demonstrate on a reasonably high number of patients that PET is largely concordant with CT for staging of HL and that the additional value of the method has an impact on the management of the patients [6].

Partridge et al. retrospectively investigated the impact of 44 pretreatment scans on the management of HL patients. PET found almost twice as many positive sites than CT (159 vs. 84) and 21 patients would have had their staging changed as a result of PET (18 upstaging and three downstaging. According to PET, treatment strategy should have been changed in 11 patients, in 10 cases to a more intensive therapy. 12 patients had a total of 19 extranodal disease sites. PEt alone detected 15 of these sites, four sites were seen on both CT and PET, and PET missed no sites seen on CT. This study suggested a very high sensitivity for detection of organ involvement [7].

Jerusalem et al. undertook the first thorough study of region-by-region accuracy in HL. They scanned 33 patients before initial treatment or before treatment of relapse and evaluated the impact on nodal staging. Overall concordant results were seen in 22 patients, but in two patients both methods indicated lesions that were not shown by the other method. In six patients, PET showed involvement of more regions than conventional methods. The sensitivities of PET for detecting involved lymph node regions were 95 % in peripheral regions, 96 % in thoracic regions, and 78 % in abdominal/pelvic regions. The corresponding sensitivities for conventional staging procedures were 80 %, 81 %, and 86 %. Although the impact on staging was clear, PET staging would only have had impact on treatment strategy in one patient [8]. Weihrauch et al. applied a quite similar approach. In 22 patients they identified 72 involved lymph node regions. In 48 lesions in 22 patients, both CT and PET were positive. 20 lesions in 11 patients were positive on PET but not detected by CT or other conventional staging methods. Sensitivity of PET and CT was 88 % and 74 %, respectively, and out of 22 patients, four were upstaged due to PET findings [9].

The general impression from these early studies was that:

1. PET seemed to have a relatively high sensitivity for nodal staging.
2. PET was clearly more sensitive than CT in detecting extranodal disease, both in the bone marrow and in other organs (Fig. 1.2).
3. PET had a consistent, large influence on the staging, with a potential impact on treatment strategy in a substantial number of patients.

More recent studies have confirmed these findings: Cerci and colleagues enrolled 210 newly diagnosed HL patients in a prospective study aiming to evaluate the cost-effectiveness of PET in HL staging. They found sensitivity for initial staging of PET was higher than that of CT in initial staging (97.9 % vs. 87.3 %). The incorporation of PET in the staging procedure upstaged disease in 50 (24 %) patients and downstaged disease in 17 (8 %) patients, with a resultant changes in treatment in 32 (15 %) patients [10].

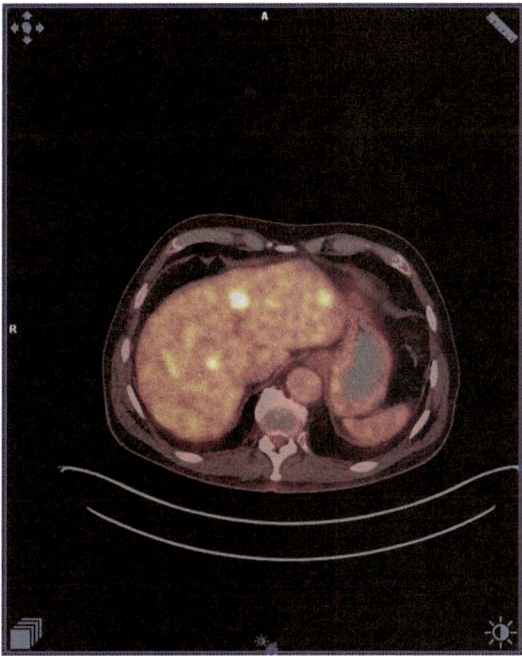

Fig. 1.2 An example of extranodal manifestation of HL in the liver, only vaguely visible on CT but with clearly pathological FDG uptake in the liver

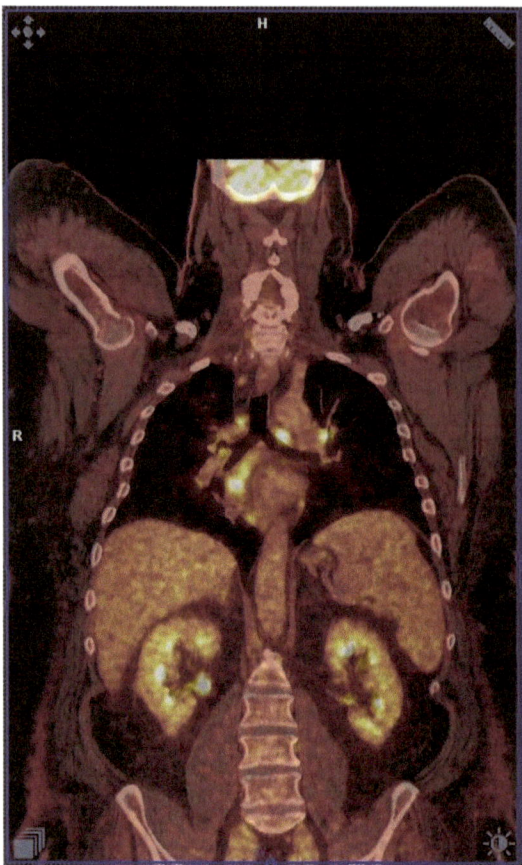

Fig. 1.3 Inflammatory FDG uptake in mediastinal lymph nodes. The pattern mimics lymphoma but was a result of a chronic lung infections

But the high sensitivity of stand-alone PET came at the expensive of a relatively large number of false positive results, in part due to well-known pitfalls including FDG uptake in reactive lymph nodes due to inflammation/infection (Figs. 1.3 and 1.4), brown fat uptake (Fig. 1.5), physiological bowel uptake, uptake due to thymic rebound, etc. After the introduction of PET/CT, such false positive findings became much less common, resulting in a high specificity despite the high sensitivity.

1.4 PET/CT Staging

The first study of PET/CT was a prospective comparison of PET, CT, and PET/CT in 99 newly diagnosed HL patients. The results of PET and PET/CT were not disclosed to the treating physicians, and furthermore, the reviewers of PET, CT, and PET/CT were blinded to the results the other imaging modalities. In nodal regions, the sensitivity of PET and PET/CT was higher than that of CT (92 % and 92 % vs. 83 %). PET had more false positive nodal sites than CT and PET/CT (1.6 % vs 0.7 % and 0.5 %). For evaluation of organs, PET and PET/CT had high sensitivities (86 % and 73 %) while CT detected only 37 % of involved organs. PET would have upstaged 19 % of patients and downstaged 5 % of patients, leading to a different treatment strategy in 9 % of patients [11]. An analysis of the same group of patients revealed that FDG avidity varied between different subtypes of classical HL and that the FDG uptake in nodular lymphocyte-predominant (NLP) HL was significantly lower than in classical HL [12].

Bednaruk-Młyński and colleagues compared the results of staging CT and PET/CT in 96 HL patients. Also in this study, the radiologists and nuclear medicine physicians were blinded to results of the other modality and to the clinical course of the patients. The number of patients with stage I, II, III, and IV disease based on CT versus PET/CT was 5 vs. 7, 49 vs. 37, 28 vs. 22, and 14 vs. 30, respectively. PET/CT changed the stage in 33 (34 %) patients; 28 % were upstaged and 6 % downstaged. Upstaging was mainly caused by detection of new extranodal involvements (47 sites in 26 patients): the bone marrow (10 patients), spleen (5 patients), and lung (2 patients). Downstaging resulted from the absence of FDG uptake in enlarged nodes (<15 mm) in the abdomen and pelvis. PET/CT led to a treatment modification in 20 (21 %) of the patients, with 16 patients allocated to more intensive treatment and 4 to less intensive treatment [13].

A different approach was taken by El-Galaly et al. who performed a historical comparison of staging patterns in Danish HL patients before and after the introduction of staging PET/CT. Their analysis covered two large cohorts of patients with classical HL staged without PET/CT ($n = 324$) and with PET/CT ($n = 406$). In PET/CT-staged patients, stage I disease was less frequent (16 % vs. 27 %) while stage IV disease was

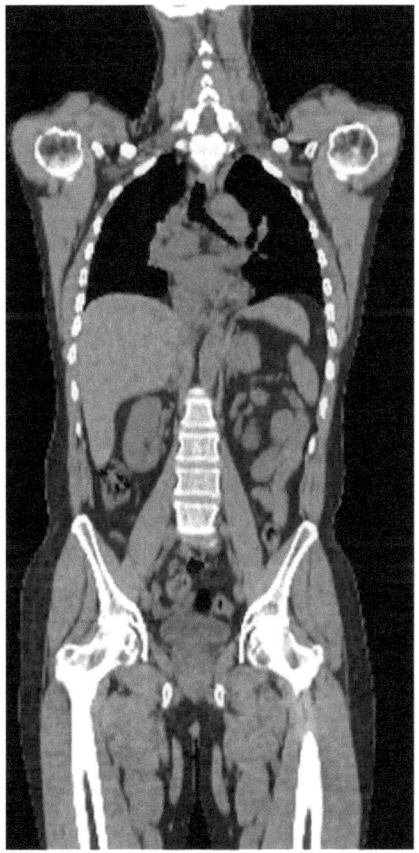
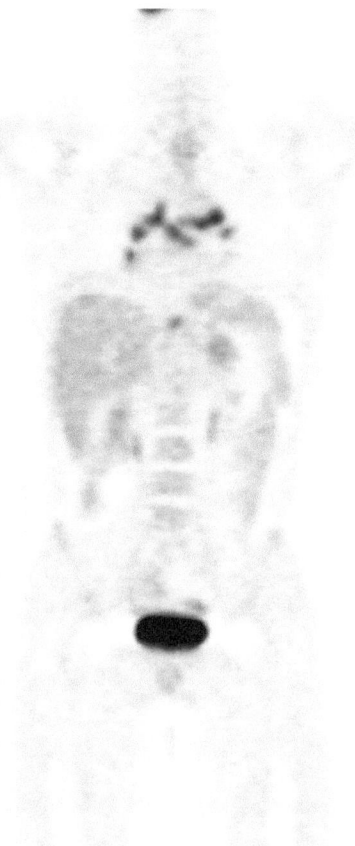

Fig. 1.4 An example of false positive PET results. Hodgkin lymphoma patient scanned 2 months after completion of treatment. PET/CT early during chemotherapy had shown a complete metabolic response. A biopsy was taken from the PET-positive mediastinal lymph nodes, and the histology showed a sarcomatoid reaction, with no signs of malignant disease

more frequent (17 % vs. 10 %). Imaging-detected skeletal involvement was recognized more often in PET/CT-staged patients (17 % vs. 2 %), and the presence of focal skeletal PET/CT lesions was associated with higher risk of progression [14].

NLP HL has more characteristics in common with indolent lymphomas, and as mentioned above this subtype has lower FDG avidity than classical Hodgkin lymphoma [12], but still the sensitivity of PET/CT staging seems to be high. In a study of 35 patients with this rare histological subtype, Grellier et al. found that PET/CT resulted in stage migration in 34 % of the patients, with detection of disease in the bone or bone marrow in 20 % of the patients. The identification of advanced disease in NLP HL is particularly important for management, since localized NLP

HL is often treated with local radiotherapy alone and thus without systemic therapy [15].

Figures 1.6 and 1.7 show PET/CT images of HL patients with stage II and stage III, respectively.

1.5   Stage Migration and Overtreatment

Hodgkin lymphoma can be cured in the vast majority of cases but cure comes the price of serious treatment-related late effects, including second cancers and cardiopulmonary disease [16]. While optimizing cure is always a goal of clinical cancer research, in first-line Hodgkin lymphoma treatment, there is a stronger call for reduction of the treatment intensity in order to avoid unneces-

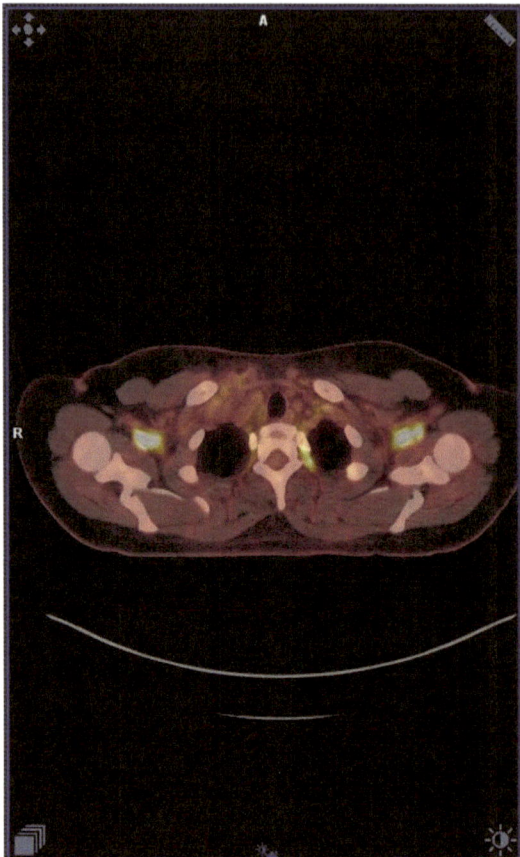

Fig. 1.5 FDG uptake in brown fat. This pitfall represented a serious challenge but after the introduction of PET/CT no longer a major cause of false positive interpretations

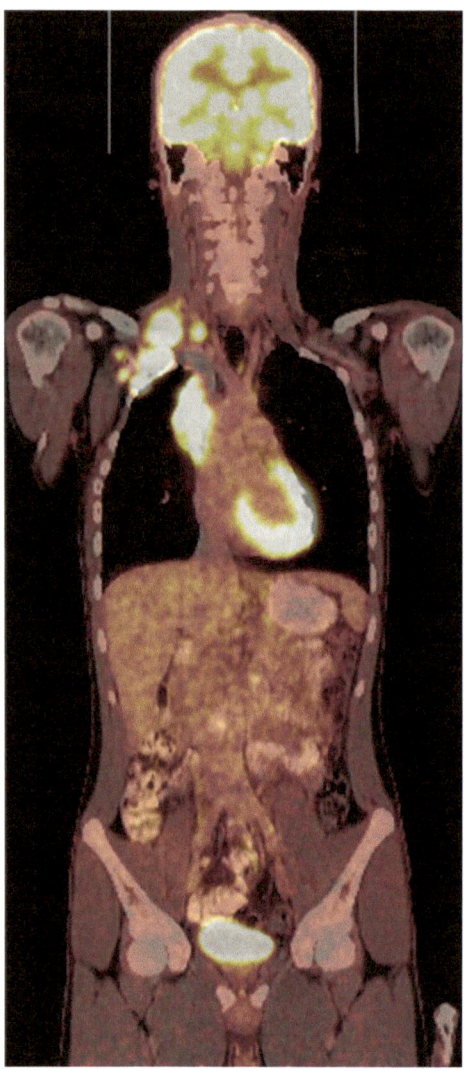

Fig. 1.6 Hodgkin lymphoma, stage II disease, with a classical distribution of involved lymph nodes in the upper mediastinum and lower neck

sary overtreatment in some patients without losing efficacy for others [17]. As discussed, PET/CT results in considerable upward stage migration and allocation of 10–20 % of patients to a more advanced treatment group. If PET/CT is incorporated into routine and the existing treatment paradigms are kept unchanged, this will result in even more overtreatment (Fig. 1.8). The introduction of more sensitive staging methods also calls for relevant therapeutic modifications, so the more refined imaging is used to individualize therapy rather than to aggravate the overtreatment problem. Such treatment modifications as a consequence of PET/CT have indeed already taken place: The shift from involved-field radiotherapy to involved-node radiotherapy resulted in

a dramatic reduction of radiation fields to HL patients, and this change was a direct result of the more accuracy baseline imaging by PET/CT [18].

1.6 Is Contrast-Enhanced CT Necessary in the PET/CT Era?

The CT part of a PET/CT scan may be performed with contrast enhancement (ceCT) at full radiation dose to obtain a high-quality CT examination

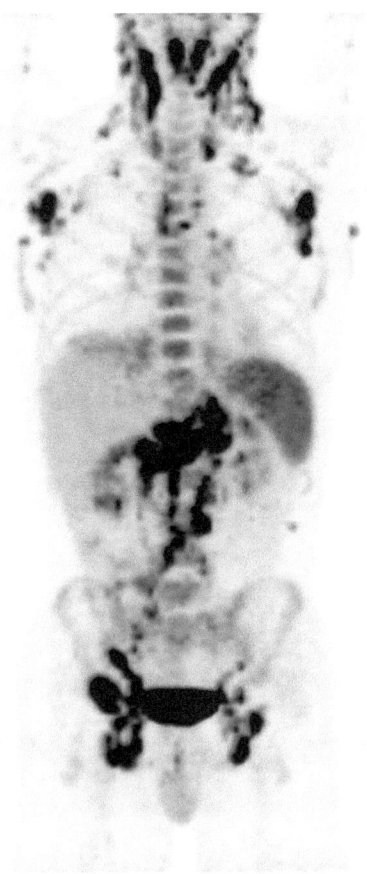

Fig. 1.7 Hodgkin lymphoma, stage III disease. Involvement of almost all lymph node regions and the spleen

or without contrast using a lower radiation dose. Low-dose CT is used to correct for the attenuation of radioactivity within the patient and to localize abnormalities seen on PET, with less radiation than a full diagnostic examination. Whichever protocol is used, CT must be acquired during shallow breathing or end of expiration to avoid misregistration and artifacts [19]. A number of studies have compared PET/CT with and without ceCT, and although ceCT may identify additional findings and improve detection of abdominal and pelvic disease, this rarely has an impact on management [20–22]. The use of contrast may result in small errors in the measurement of FDG uptake due to an effect on attenuation correction; this may cause errors in comparison of uptake between tumor and refer-

ence sites by causing FDG uptake to be overestimated in the mediastinum and liver by 10–15 %. Although these errors are unlikely to be clinically important for staging purposes, they may be important for response assessment during and after treatment [23, 24]. In practice, many patients have already undergone a ceCT as part of the diagnostic workup and before referral to PET/CT. If performed, it is recommended that ceCT be performed during a single visit in combination with PET/CT.

1.7 The Need for Bone Marrow Biopsy

The Cotswold modifications to the Ann Arbor classification discouraged all invasive staging procedures with exception of bone marrow biopsy in selected patients [4]. While stand-alone CT is insufficient for evaluation of HL infiltration in the bone marrow, PET/CT detects areas of pathological skeletal FDG uptake suggestive of bone marrow involvement (BMI) in 10–20 % of the patients. PET-detected BMI is usually seen as areas of focally increased FDG uptake and often without accompanying morphological changes on CT [25–28] (Fig. 1.9). The fact that these lesions are seen in up to one-fifth of the patients has changed the old perception of bone marrow involvement being rare in HL. Most studies relying on bone marrow biopsy for detection of BMI only report frequencies of around 5–8 % for BMI in HL [29, 30]. The use of iliac crest bone marrow biopsy as a surrogate for the whole bone marrow compartment has been challenged by frequent finding of focal FDG lesions in the bone marrow in patients undergoing PET/CT staging. In addition, one-sided bone marrow involvement has been reported in nearly half of the HL patients undergoing bilateral bone marrow biopsies [31]. Directed biopsies and/or additional imaging with scintigraphy and MRI has supported the presence of HL in areas of otherwise unexplained focal FDG uptake in the bone marrow [21, 27]. Furthermore, there seems to be complete agreement between FDG uptake in the site of the bone marrow biopsy and results

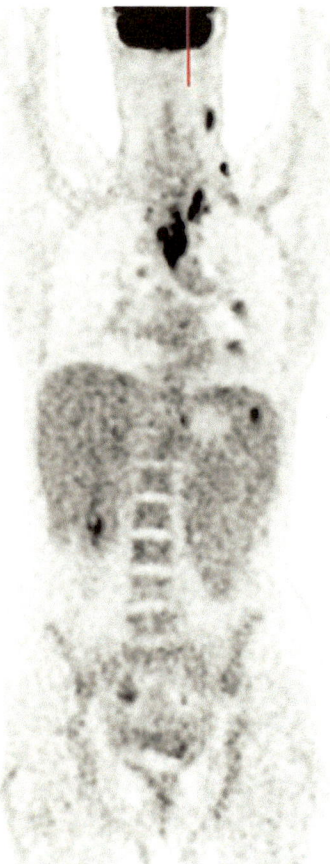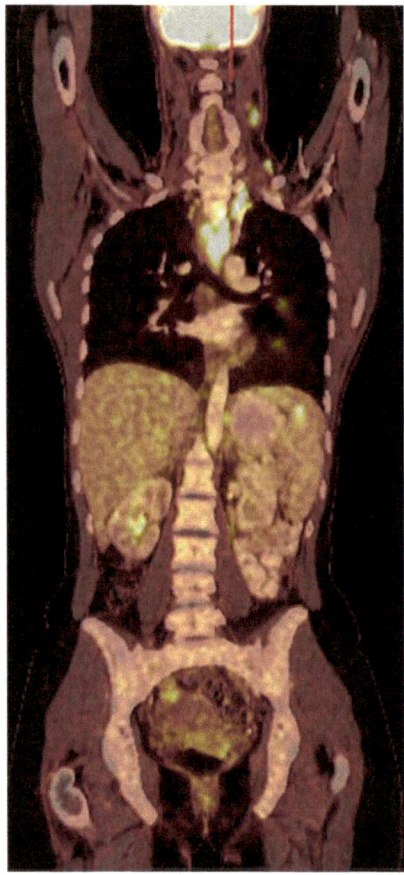

Fig. 1.8 Upward stage migration as a consequence of PET/CT. This young lady was diagnosed with classical Hodgkin lymphoma and stage IIA disease according to CT performed before referral. Staging PET/CT showed a clearly PET-positive lesion in the spleen. There was no corresponding abnormality on CT and biopsy was not feasible. The original treatment plan was changed from a brief course of chemotherapy followed by local irradia-tion to the neck and upper mediastinum to 6 cycles of combination chemotherapy. During her treatment, she developed pneumonitis as a result of bleomycin treatment, and she needed high-dose prednisone treatment for several months. With the patient well and in continued remission more than 5 years after treatment, it is still not clear if PET/CT saved her from undertreatment or resulted in overtreatment

of bone marrow biopsy [32]. In conclusion, PET/CT has much higher sensitivity for bone marrow involvement than conventional bone marrow biopsy [33]. The few patients with BMI initially not detected by PET/CT but only by routine bone marrow biopsy almost exclusively present with advanced-stage disease based on the PET/CT findings, and therefore the added diagnostic information from bone marrow biopsies very rarely leads to changes in clinical management [25, 26]. The presence of diffuse FDG uptake throughout the whole axial skeleton without simultaneous focal lesions is a common finding in patients with newly diagnosed HL (Fig. 1.10). Despite FDG uptake at the sites of bone marrow biopsies, patients with this kind of diffuse FDG uptake in the bone marrow usually (but not always) present with negative bone marrow biopsies [25, 28, 34, 35]. Other findings suggest that inflammatory response may explain the diffuse FDG uptake in the bone marrow of HL patients since anemia and increased leukocyte count are associated with the presence of a diffuse FDG uptake [5, 17, 25, 36] Finally, a study

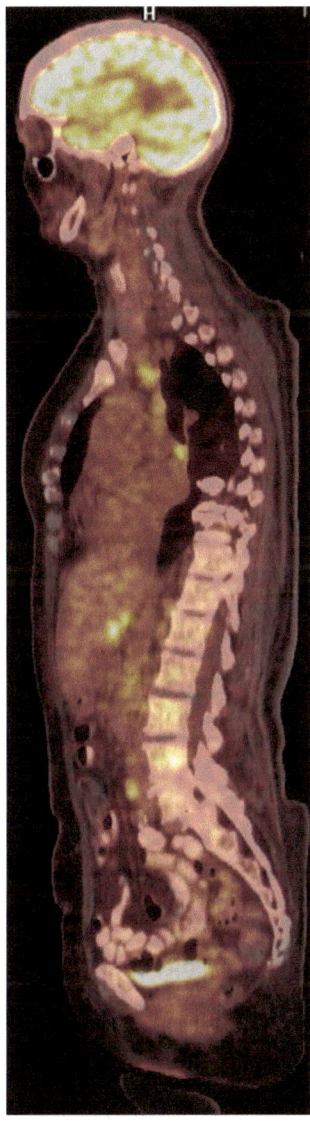

Fig. 1.10 Stage II disease with heavy disease burden and diffusely increased uptake in the bone marrow

1.8   Newer PET Tracers

Fig. 1.9 Focally increased FDG uptake in the bone marrow of lumbar vertebrae, without accompanying morphological changes on CT

has shown that there is a high degree of concordance in the reporting of PET/CT-ascertained bone marrow involvement [36]. The Lugano classification acknowledges the insignificant contribution of routine bone marrow biopsy to the baseline staging of HL by recommending against its use in PET/CT-staged HL patients [19, 37]. Thus, the last reminiscence of the pathological staging included in the original Ann Arbor classification has finally been eliminated.

Like other cancers, HL is characterized by deregulated cell cycle progression and most anticancer drugs are designed to inhibit cell proliferation. So a tracer enabling imaging of cell proliferation could be useful for both initial characterization and treatment monitoring of the disease. FDG uptake is somewhat correlated with cell proliferation, but this correlation is weakened by a number of factors, including FDG uptake in nonmalignant lesions [38, 39]. The nucleoside [^{11}C]thymidine was the first PET tracer to specifically address cell proliferation. Early studies showed that [^{11}C]thymidine could determine both disease extent and early response to chemotherapy in aggressive non-Hodgkin lymphoma (NHL) patients [40, 41].

However, the short 20 min half-life of ^{11}C along with rapid in vivo metabolism has limited the clinical application of [^{11}C]thymidine. The thymidine analogue 3′-deoxy-3′-[^{18}F]fluorothymidine (FLT) offers a more suitable half-life of 110 min (same as FDG) and is stable in vivo [42]. More recent studies have shown that FLT-PET can sensitively identify lymphoma sites [43]. FLT uptake is highly correlated with proliferation rate and may thus be able to distinguish between high- and low-grade lymphomas [44, 45]. And furthermore, recent studies have showed a potential of FLT for imaging early response to treatment in lymphoma [46–49]. Amino acid metabolism of cancer cells is influenced by catabolic processes favoring tumor growth [50]. It has been shown that increased uptake of amino acids reflects the increased transport and protein synthesis of malignant tissue [51, 52]. This is the background for PET imaging of amino acid metabolism with the labeled amino acids L-[methyl-^{11}C]methionine (MET) and O-2-[^{18}F]fluoroethyl)-L-tyrosine (FET) [53]. Nuutinen et al. studied 32 lymphoma patients and found MET-PET highly sensitive for the detection of disease sites although there was no correlation between MET uptake and patient outcome [54]. While these results are encouraging, it should be noted that no studies have shown the usefulness or cost-effectiveness of amino acid or nucleoside tracers in large patient cohorts. Furthermore, high physiological tracer uptake in the abdomen limits the usefulness of these tracers for imaging of abdominal and pelvic lymphomas.

1.9 International Guidelines and the Lugano Classification

In recent years, several national and regional guidelines have included PET/CT in the recommended HL staging workup [55]. Recently, a revision of the international recommendations for staging and response assessment of lymphoma was published (the Lugano classification) [37]. These recommendations are accompanied by internationally accepted guidelines for the use of imaging in lymphoma [19]. Both the imaging

recommendations and the staging guidelines recommend PET/CT for routine staging and response assessment of HL, and in patients with PET/CT staging, routine BMB is discouraged, based on the data presented above. The Lugano classification has abandoned the use of B symptoms (fever, night sweats, weight loss) as signs of disseminated disease in NHL, since these constitutional symptoms do not confer an unfavorable outcome according to the different NHL prognostic indices [56–58]. However, since the presence of one or more B symptoms is a prognostic factor in HL which still plays a role in treatment allocation, HL patients continue to be categorized into stages I–IV (primarily according to PET/CT) and with the suffix A or B (with or without B symptoms). In the imaging recommendations it is acknowledged that a 4-point staging classification is a rather crude representation of the modern, advanced imaging methods. Modern CT and PET methodology allows for advanced quantification of both anatomical and metabolic image information, and it is encouraged to explore the value of such quantitative measures in the near future. In a few years, the disease stage may very well be expressed as a precise volume and a metabolic intensity rather than as a number on a four-step scale.

References

1. Engert A, Diehl V, Franklin J, Lohri A, Dorken B, Ludwig WD, et al. Escalated-dose BEACOPP in the treatment of patients with advanced-stage Hodgkin's lymphoma: 10 years of follow-up of the GHSG HD9 study. J Clin Oncol. 2009;27(27):4548–54.
2. Engert A, Plutschow A, Eich HT, Lohri A, Dorken B, Borchmann P, et al. Reduced treatment intensity in patients with early-stage Hodgkin's lymphoma. N Engl J Med. 2010;363(7):640–52.
3. Carbone PP, Kaplan HS, Musshoff K, Smithers DW, Tubiana M. Report of the Committee on Hodgkin's Disease Staging Classification. Cancer Res. 1971;31(11):1860–1.
4. Lister TA, Crowther D, Sutcliffe SB, Glatstein E, Canellos GP, Young RC, et al. Report of a committee convened to discuss the evaluation and staging of patients with Hodgkin's disease: Cotswolds meeting. J Clin Oncol. 1989;7(11):1630–6.
5. Weiler-Sagie M, Bushelev O, Epelbaum R, Dann EJ, Haim N, Avivi I, et al. (18)F-FDG avidity in lymphoma

readdressed: a study of 766 patients. J Nucl Med. 2010;51(1):25–30.

6. Bangerter M, Moog F, Buchmann I, Kotzerke J, Griesshammer M, Hafner M, et al. Whole-body 2-[18F]-fluoro-2-deoxy-D-glucose positron emission tomography (FDG-PET) for accurate staging of Hodgkin's disease. Ann Oncol. 1998;9(10):1117–22.

7. Partridge S, Timothy A, O'Doherty MJ, Hain SF, Rankin S, Mikhaeel G. 2-Fluorine-18-fluoro-2-deoxy-D glucose positron emission tomography in the pretreatment staging of Hodgkin's disease: influence on patient management in a single institution. Ann Oncol. 2000;11(10):1273–9.

8. Jerusalem G, Beguin Y, Fassotte MF, Najjar F, Paulus P, Rigo P, et al. Whole-body positron emission tomography using 18F-fluorodeoxyglucose compared to standard procedures for staging patients with Hodgkin's disease. Haematologica. 2001; 86(3):266–73.

9. Weihrauch MR, Re D, Bischoff S, Dietlein M, Scheidhauer K, Krug B, et al. Whole-body positron emission tomography using 18F-fluorodeoxyglucose for initial staging of patients with Hodgkin's disease. Ann Hematol. 2002;81(1):20–5.

10. Cerci JJ, Trindade E, Buccheri V, Fanti S, Coutinho AMN, Zanoni L, et al. Consistency of FDG-PET accuracy and cost-effectiveness in initial staging of patients with Hodgkin lymphoma across jurisdictions. Clin Lymphoma Myeloma Leuk. 2011;11(4):314–20.

11. Hutchings M, Loft A, Hansen M, Pedersen LM, Berthelsen AK, Keiding S, et al. Position emission tomography with or without computed tomography in the primary staging of Hodgkin's lymphoma. Haematologica. 2006;91(4):482–9.

12. Hutchings M, Loft A, Hansen M, Ralfkiaer E, Specht L. Different histopathological subtypes of Hodgkin lymphoma show significantly different levels of FDG uptake. Hematol Oncol. 2006;24(3):146–50.

13. Bednaruk-Młyński E, Pieńkowska J, Skórzak A, Małkowski B, Kulikowski W, Subocz E, et al. Comparison of positron emission tomography/computed tomography with classical contrast-enhanced computed tomography in the initial staging of Hodgkin lymphoma. Leuk Lymphoma. 2014;56(2):377–82.

14. El Galaly TC, Hutchings M, Mylam KJ, Brown Pde N, Bukh A, Johnsen HE, et al. Impact of 18F-fluorodeoxyglucose positron emission tomography/computed tomography staging in newly diagnosed classical Hodgkin lymphoma: fewer cases with stage I disease and more with skeletal involvement. Leuk Lymphoma. 2014;55(10):2349–55.

15. Grellier J, Vercellino L, Leblanc T, Merlet P, Thieblemont C, Weinmann P, et al. Performance of FDG PET/CT at initial diagnosis in a rare lymphoma: nodular lymphocyte-predominant Hodgkin lymphoma. Eur J Nucl Med Mol Imaging. 2014;41(11):2023–30.

16. Aleman BM, van den Belt-Dusebout AW, Klokman WJ, Van't Veer MB, Bartelink H, van Leeuwen FE. Long-term cause-specific mortality of patients treated for Hodgkin's disease. J Clin Oncol. 2003;21(18):3431–9.

17. Hutchings M. How does PET/CT help in selecting therapy for patients with Hodgkin lymphoma? ASH Educ Program Book. 2012;2012(1):322–7.

18. Girinsky T, van der Maazen R, Specht L, Aleman B, Poortmans P, Lievens Y, et al. Involved-node radiotherapy (INRT) in patients with early Hodgkin lymphoma: concepts and guidelines. Radiother Oncol. 2006;79(3):270–7.

19. Barrington SF, Mikhaeel NG, Kostakoglu L, Meignan M, Hutchings M, Mueller SP, et al. Role of imaging in the staging and response assessment of lymphoma: consensus of the International Conference on Malignant Lymphomas Imaging Working Group. J Clin Oncol. 2014;32(27):3048–58.

20. Chiaravalloti A, Danieli R, Caracciolo CR, Travascio L, Cantonetti M, Gallamini A, et al. Initial staging of Hodgkin's disease: role of contrast-enhanced 18F FDG PET/CT. Medicine. 2014;93(8), e50.

21. Schaefer NG, Hany TF, Taverna C, Seifert B, Stumpe KDM, von Schulthess GK, et al. Non-Hodgkin lymphoma and Hodgkin disease: coregistered FDG PET and CT at staging and restaging – do we need contrast-enhanced CT? Radiology. 2004;232(3):823–9.

22. Chalaye J, Luciani A, Enache C, Beaussart P, Lhermite C, Evangelista E, et al. Clinical impact of contrast-enhanced computed tomography combined with low-dose 18F-fluorodeoxyglucose positron emission tomography/computed tomography on routine lymphoma patient management. Leuk Lymphoma. 2014;55(12):2887–92.

23. Vriens D, Visser E, de Geus-Oei L-F, Oyen W. Methodological considerations in quantification of oncological FDG PET studies. Eur J Nucl Med Mol Imaging. 2010;37(7):1408–25.

24. Berthelsen AK, Holm S, Loft A, Klausen TL, Andersen F, Højgaard L. PET/CT with intravenous contrast can be used for PET attenuation correction in cancer patients. Eur J Nucl Med Mol Imaging. 2005;32(10):1167–75.

25. El Galaly TC, d'Amore F, Mylam KJ, Nully Brown P, Bøgsted M, Bukh A, et al. Routine bone marrow biopsy has little or no therapeutic consequence for positron emission tomography/computed tomography-staged treatment-naive patients with Hodgkin lymphoma. J Clin Oncol. 2012;30(36):4508–14.

26. Weiler-Sagie M, Kagna O, Dann E, Ben Barak A, Israel O. Characterizing bone marrow involvement in Hodgkin's lymphoma by FDG-PET/CT. Eur J Nucl Med Mol Imaging. 2014;41(6):1133–40.

27. Purz S, Mauz-Körholz C, Körholz D, Hasenclever D, Krausse A, Sorge I, et al. [18F]fluorodeoxyglucose positron emission tomography for detection of bone marrow involvement in children and adolescents with Hodgkin's lymphoma. J Clin Oncol. 2011;29(26):3523–8.

28. Chen-Liang TH, Martin-Santos T, Jerez A, Senent L, Orero MT, Remigia MJ, et al. The role of bone marrow biopsy and FDG-PET/CT in identifying bone

marrow infiltration in the initial diagnosis of high grade non-Hodgkin B-cell lymphoma and Hodgkin lymphoma. accuracy in a multicenter series of 372 patients. Am J Hematol. 2015;90(8):686–90.

29. Howell SJ, Grey M, Chang J, Morgenstern GR, Cowan RA, Deakin DP, et al. The value of bone marrow examination in the staging of Hodgkin's lymphoma: a review of 955 cases seen in a regional cancer centre. Br J Haematol. 2002;119(2):408–11.

30. Levis A, Pietrasanta D, Godio L, Vitolo U, Ciravegna G, Di Vito F, et al. A large-scale study of bone marrow involvement in patients with Hodgkin's lymphoma. Clin Lymphoma. 2004;5(1):50–5.

31. BRUNNING RD, BLOOMFIELD CD, McKENNA RW, PETERSON L. Bilateral trephine bone marrow biopsies in lymphoma and other neoplastic diseases. Ann Intern Med. 1975;82(3):365–6.

32. Adams H, Kwee T, Fijnheer R, Dubois S, Nievelstein R, de Klerk J. Bone marrow FDG-PET/CT in Hodgkin lymphoma revisited: do imaging and pathology match? Ann Nucl Med. 2015;29(2):132–7.

33. Adams HJA, Kwee TC, de Keizer B, Fijnheer R, de Klerk JMH, Littooij AS, et al. Systematic review and meta-analysis on the diagnostic performance of FDG-PET/CT in detecting bone marrow involvement in newly diagnosed Hodgkin lymphoma: is bone marrow biopsy still necessary? Ann Oncol. 2014;25(5):921–7.

34. Adams HJA, Kwee TC, Fijnheer R, Dubois SV, Nievelstein RAJ, de Klerk JMH. Diffusely increased bone marrow FDG uptake in recently untreated lymphoma: incidence and relevance. Eur J Haematol. 2015;95(1):83–9.

35. Chiang SB, Rebenstock A, Guan L, Alavi A, Zhuang H. Diffuse bone marrow involvement of Hodgkin lymphoma mimics hematopoietic cytokine-mediated FDG uptake on FDG PET imaging. Clin Nucl Med. 2003;28(8):674–6.

36. Zwarthoud C, Ouvier M, Borra A, Bergesio F, Chauvie S, Biggi A, et al. Patterns of PET/CT-assessed bone-marrow involvement in newly diagnosed Hodgkin lymphoma; a detailed review of 150 ABVD treated patients. Leuk Lymphoma. 2015;56:1233. Ref Type: Abstract.

37. Cheson BD, Fisher RI, Barrington SF, Cavalli F, Schwartz LH, Zucca E, et al. Recommendations for initial evaluation, staging, and response assessment of Hodgkin and Non-Hodgkin lymphoma: the Lugano classification. J Clin Oncol. 2014;32(27):3059–68.

38. Buck AK, Halter G, Schirrmeister H, Kotzerke J, Wurziger I, Glatting G, et al. Imaging proliferation in lung tumors with PET: 18F-FLT versus 18F-FDG. J Nucl Med. 2003;44(9):1426–31.

39. Sandherr M, von Schilling C, Link T, Stock K, von Bubnoff N, Peschel C, et al. Pitfalls in imaging Hodgkin's disease with computed tomography and positron emission tomography using fluorine-18-fluorodeoxyglucose. Ann Oncol. 2001;12(5):719–22.

40. Martiat P, Ferrant A, Labar D, Cogneau M, Bol A, Michel C, et al. In vivo measurement of carbon-11 thymidine uptake in non-Hodgkin's lymphoma using positron emission tomography. J Nucl Med. 1988;29(10):1633–7.

41. Shields AF, Mankoff DA, Link JM, Graham MM, Eary JF, Kozawa SM, et al. Carbon-11-thymidine and FDG to measure therapy response. J Nucl Med. 1998;39(10):1757–62.

42. Shields AF, Grierson JR, Dohmen BM, Machulla HJ, Stayanoff JC, Lawhorn-Crews JM, et al. Imaging proliferation in vivo with [F-18]FLT and positron emission tomography. Nat Med. 1998;4(11):1334–6.

43. Buchmann I, Neumaier B, Schreckenberger M, Reske S. [18F]3′-deoxy-3′-fluorothymidine-PET in NHL patients: whole-body biodistribution and imaging of lymphoma manifestations--a pilot study. Cancer Biother Radiopharm. 2004;19(4):436–42.

44. Buck AK, Bommer M, Stilgenbauer S, Juweid M, Glatting G, Schirrmeister H, et al. Molecular imaging of proliferation in malignant lymphoma. Cancer Res. 2006;66(22):11055–61.

45. Kasper B, Egerer G, Gronkowski M, Haufe S, Lehnert T, Eisenhut M, et al. Functional diagnosis of residual lymphomas after radiochemotherapy with positron emission tomography comparing FDG- and FLT-PET. Leuk Lymphoma. 2007;48(4):746–53.

46. Buck AK, Kratochwil C, Glatting G, Juweid M, Bommer M, Tepsic D, et al. Early assessment of therapy response in malignant lymphoma with the thymidine analogue [18F]FLT. Eur J Nucl Med Mol Imaging. 2007;34(11):1775–82.

47. Herrmann K, Buck AK, Schuster T, Rudelius M, Wester HJ, Graf N, et al. A pilot study to evaluate 3′-deoxy-3′-18F-fluorothymidine PET for initial and early response imaging in mantle cell lymphoma. J Nucl Med. 2011;52(12):1898–902.

48. Herrmann K, Buck AK, Schuster T, Junger A, Wieder H, Graf N, et al. Predictive value of initial 18F-FLT uptake in patients with aggressive non-Hodgkin lymphoma receiving R-CHOP treatment. J Nucl Med. 2011;52(5):690–6.

49. Graf N, Herrmann K, den Hollander J, Fend F, Schuster T, Wester HJ, et al. Imaging proliferation to monitor early response of lymphoma to cytotoxic treatment. Mol Imaging Biol. 2008;10(6):349–55.

50. Hoffman RM. Altered methionine metabolism, DNA methylation and oncogene expression in carcinogenesis. A review and synthesis. Biochim Biophys Acta. 1984;738(1-2):49–87.

51. Stern PH, Wallace CD, Hoffman RM. Altered methionine metabolism occurs in all members of a set of diverse human tumor cell lines. J Cell Physiol. 1984;119(1):29–34.

52. Wheatley DN. On the problem of linear incorporation of amino acids into cell protein. Experientia. 1982;38(7):818–20.

53. Leskinen-Kallio S, Ruotsalainen U, Nagren K, Teras M, Joensuu H. Uptake of carbon-11-methionine and fluorodeoxyglucose in non-Hodgkin's lymphoma: a PET study. J Nucl Med. 1991;32(6):1211–8.

54. Nuutinen J, Leskinen S, Lindholm P, Soderstrom KO, Nagren K, Huhtala S, et al. Use of carbon-11 methio-

nine positron emission tomography to assess malignancy grade and predict survival in patients with lymphomas. Eur J Nucl Med. 1998;25(7):729–35.

55. Eichenauer DA, Engert A, André M, Federico M, Illidge T, Hutchings M, et al. Hodgkin's lymphoma: ESMO Clinical Practice Guidelines for diagnosis, treatment and follow-up. Ann Oncol. 2014;25 suppl 3:iii70–5.

56. A predictive model for aggressive non-Hodgkin's lymphoma. The International Non-Hodgkin's Lymphoma Prognostic Factors Project. N Engl J Med. 1993;329(14):987–94.

57. Solal-Celigny P, Roy P, Colombat P, White J, Armitage JO, Arranz-Saez R, et al. Follicular lymphoma international prognostic index. Blood. 2004;104(5):1258–65.

58. Hoster E, Dreyling M, Klapper W, Gisselbrecht C, van Hoof A, Kluin-Nelemans HC, et al. A new prognostic index (MIPI) for patients with advanced-stage mantle cell lymphoma. Blood. 2008;111(2):558–65.

Josée M. Zijlstra and Pieter G. Raijmakers

2.1 Introduction

Hodgkin lymphoma is relatively rare disease, with an annual incidence of 3 per 100,000. The peak incidence is in the early adulthood and in the elderly. Patients most commonly present with lymphadenopathy in the cervical region and the mediastinum. The mediastinal region often shows bulky disease. When more regions are involved, the areas are usually contiguous, consistent with the view that spread is predominantly through the lymphatic channels [1]. Accurate staging and restaging provide important prognostic information and dictate the appropriate treatment strategy. With the introduction of FDG-PET and later on of FDG-PET/CT during the last decennia, the accuracy of staging and restaging has improved enormously [2, 3].

The widely used International Working Group criteria for response assessment of lymphoma, published in 1999, were based predominantly on CT and did not include PET as part of response assessment [4]. The term "complete remission unconfirmed" (CRu) was originally coined to describe persistence of a residual mass post-therapy, with resolution of all clinical symptoms. Patients with Hodgkin lymphoma often present with a bulky mediastinal mass, while after treatment fibrotic residual tissue can be observed. An optimal treatment strategy for patients with HL combines high cure rates with minimal toxicity. The correct identification of patients with a complete remission, with or without large residual masses, reduces the number of patients exposed to unnecessary toxicity. With the introduction of FDG, the ability to distinguish between viable tumor and necrosis or fibrosis became available [5]. In one study, it was observed that that the majority of the CRu patients had negative FDG-PET findings with progression-free survival rates equivalent with CR patients [6]. Hence, FDG-PET may be useful in finding the balance between a highly effective treatment and minimal toxicity. Considering the more widespread use of FDG-PET in response assessment of lymphoma, it became clear that the International Working Group criteria warranted revision. For this purpose, in 2007 the Competence Network Malignant Lymphoma convened an International Harmonization Project with five subcommittees among which the imaging subcommittee. The aim was to develop guidelines for performing and interpreting FDG-PET for treatment assessment in lymphoma, to ensure the reliability of the method, both in the context of clinical trials and in clinical practice. Since the publication of the revised Cheson criteria for staging and restaging in malignant lymphoma [7, 8], PET has

J.M. Zijlstra, MD, PhD (✉)
Department of Hematology, VU University Medical Center, De Boelelaan 1117, 1081HV Amsterdam, The Netherlands
e-mail: j.zijlstra@vumc.nl

P.G. Raijmakers, MD, PhD
Department of Radiology and Nuclear Medicine, VU University Medical Center, De Boelelaan 1117, 1081HV Amsterdam, The Netherlands
e-mail: p.raijmakers@vumc.nl

become a mandatory and essential diagnostic technique in evaluation treatment response. Since that time, many reports have shown the value of PET imaging of Hodgkin lymphoma for evaluation response assessment after chemotherapy or radiotherapy [9–15]. However, with increasingly sensitive and specific technologies for disease assessment by the introduction of new PET/CT imaging, a modernization of the response criteria became necessary. In 2014, the Lugano classification has been published, aiming to improve the evaluation of patients with lymphoma and enhance the ability to compare outcomes of clinical trials [16, 17]. This chapter will summarize the use of FDG-PET/CT for response evaluation after therapy and discuss the some technical considerations and pitfalls that may influence correct assessment of PET/CT. Also standardization of the interpretation of criteria and semiquantitative evaluation are being described.

2.2 Relevance of Response Monitoring

As Hodgkin lymphoma is generally a curable disease, the goal of treatment is to achieve a complete remission (CR), which is a prerequisite for cure. Accurate remission assessment after the completion of therapy is therefore essential to detect patients with incomplete response, to improve the prognosis of those patients by timely introduction of more effective treatment options. However, also overtreatment must be prevented to avoid treatment-related toxicity. As Hodgkin lymphoma patients often present with bulky lymphadenopathy, it is well know that many patients have (minor) lymphadenopathy after therapy. Particularly for response assessment at therapy conclusion, FDG-PET has been shown to be considerably more accurate than CT because of its ability to distinguish between viable tumor and necrosis or fibrosis in post-therapy residual masses that are frequently present in patients with Hodgkin lymphoma without any other clinical or biochemical evidence of disease [3]. Its routine use has been recommended to assess the post-therapy response of HL, especially if CT reveals a residual mass.

2.3 Evaluation After First-Line Therapy

During the last 20 years, many retrospective and prospective studies have been published on the value of FDG-PET and PET/CT response assessment at conclusion of therapy [9–15].

Two systematic reviews have analyzed the diagnostic accuracy of FDG-PET for posttreatment evaluation of Hodgkin lymphoma patients after first-line chemotherapy [18, 19]. Although there is a major methodological variability between the studies included in both reviews, these studies consistently show that FDG-PET has a high specificity in this setting for a pooled sensitivity (vs. the gold standard of tumor-positive biopsy/clinical follow-up of at least 1 year) of 84 % for Hodgkin lymphoma (see Table 2.1). The negative predictive value (NPV) for FDG-PET in post-therapy evaluation of HL appeared to be very high, ranging from 71 to 100 %. However, the positive predictive value (PPV) exhibits a wider range (13–100 %) with a weighted average of 62 %. Possible explanations for this relatively low PPV are the substantial fraction of HL patients that received radiation therapy prior to undergoing FDG-PET, resulting in frequent occurrence of false-positive post-radiation inflammatory changes and the more frequent

Table 2.1 Several studies have investigated the Positive Predictive value (PPV) and Negative Predictive value (NPV), illustrating the high NPV and variable PPV

Study and year	% PET positive	% PET negative	PPV (%)	NPV (%)
Filmont, 2004	44	56	78	100
Friedberg, 2004	25	75	50	96
Guay, 2003	25	75	92	92
Jerusalem, 1999, 2003	13	87	100	92
Kobe, 2008	26	74	–[a]	94
Mikosch, 2003	61	39	89	100
Mocikova, 2004	32	68	13	100
Rigacci, 2005	29	71	50	100
Schaefer, 2004	22	78	100	71
Spaepen, 2001	8	92	100	91
Wickmann, 2003	52	48	60	91

Modified from Juweid, *JNM*, [40]

[a]PET-positive patients received radiotherapy

occurrence of thymic hyperplasia in the generally younger HL patients, which can also lead to a false-positive interpretation of posttreatment PET scans. Hence, radiotherapy may hamper the interpretation of posttreatment PET scans. Recently, Morbelli et al [20] demonstrated that previous radiotherapy was the most important predictor of false-positive FDG-PET performed in asymptomatic lymphoma patients in remission. With a positive PET scan rate of about 30 % and a PPV of 62 %, misclassification of disease status due to a positive post-therapy PET affects approximately 11 % of all patients. If further treatment based on residual metabolically active disease on PET/CT is being considered, either biopsy or follow-up scan is advised. On the other hand, a 70 % frequency of negative PET combined with a NPV of 94 % translates into a misclassification of only 4 % of all patients. Even in case of a large residual mass, a biopsy is not advised [21].

Alternatively, a CT scan may offer additional information in the posttreatment evaluation of HL. Assessment of tumor size reduction on CT has been studied by Kobe et al. in their HD15 trial in advanced HL. In the subgroup of the 54 PET-positive patients with a relative reduction of less than 40 % on CT, the risk of progression or relapse within the first year was 23.1 %, compared with 5.3 % for patients with a larger reduction. So patients with HL who have PET-positive residual disease after chemotherapy and poor tumor shrinkage are at higher risk of progression or relapse [22]. Hence, a diagnostic CT scan, performed with intravenous and oral contrast agents, should also be performed.

2.4   Evaluation After Second-Line Therapy, Before Autologous Stem Cell Transplantation

For relapsed HL, reinduction chemotherapy and autologous stem cell transplantation can yield a 5-year event-free survival up to 50 % [23, 24]. However, the success of this highly toxic treatment relies on tumor chemosensitivity. Various studies [25–27] have reported that PET/CT using FDG is

prognostic in patients with relapsed or refractory HL after salvage chemotherapy before high-dose chemotherapy and autologous stem cell transplantation (ASCT) and is superior to CT alone. Three-year progression-free survival (PFS) and event-free survival (EFS) rates of 31–41 % have been reported for patients with PET-positive scans, compared with 75–82 % for patients with PET-negative scans. A meta-analysis also demonstrated a strong correlation between pre-ASCT FDG-PET results and the outcome after ASCT. A negative pre-ASCT PET not only indicated a longer PFS but also a significant gain in overall survival [28].

2.5   Visual Versus Semi-quantitative Assessment of PET/CT

Visual assessment alone appears to be adequate for determining whether PET is positive or negative at the conclusion of therapy, and quantitative or semi-quantitative approaches (e.g., using the standardized uptake value [SUV]) do not seem necessary for daily practice use. In the Lugano classification, the 5-point scale (5-PS) or Deauville score is recommended (see Table 2.2) [17]. The 5-PS was intended as a simple, reproducible scoring method, with the flexibility to change the threshold between good or poor response according to the clinical context and/or treatment strategy. The 5-PS has been validated for use at interim response assessment and was adopted as the preferred reporting method at the First International Workshop on PET in

Table 2.2 Deauville score or 5-point score for grading FDG-uptake

The *5-point score* scores the most intense uptake in a site of initial disease, if present, as follows:
1. No uptake
2. Uptake ≤ mediastinum
3. Uptake > mediastinum but ≤ liver
4. Uptake moderately higher than liver
5. Uptake markedly higher than liver and/or new lesions
X. New areas of uptake unlikely to be related to lymphoma

Lymphoma in Deauville, France (i.e., Deauville criteria), and in several international trials. At the end of treatment, residual metabolic disease with a score of 4 or 5 represents treatment failure even if uptake has reduced from baseline [16]. A score of 4 or 5 with intensity that does not change or even increases from baseline and/or new foci compatible with lymphoma represents treatment failure at the end-of-treatment assessment. However, validation of DS for end-of-treatment assessment has only been published for primary mediastinal B-cell lymphoma (PMBCL) which has similarities with mediastinal bulky HL [29].

Metabolic changes measured by standard uptake values are continuous, reflecting an in vivo therapy response scale. However, SUV measurements heavily depend on several factors related to PET protocols, e.g., interval between injection and scanning, blood glucose concentrations, body weight, and individual scanner-dependent features [30]. The variability of SUV values decreases the potential accuracy of absolute cutoff values. Hence, in daily practice, visual assessment of posttreatment PET in HL is preferred above a semiquantitative approach.

However, not only the correct scoring of the FDG avidity compared to the mediastinum and liver is important, the most relevant issue is the interpretation of these images in the clinical context. For experienced nuclear medicine physicians, the recognition of specific patterns in FDG uptake is essential [31, 32].

Most common causes of false-positive FDG-PET results in treatment evaluation are pneumonia and other infections (induced by neutropenic periods after chemotherapy), sarcoidosis and sarcoid-like reactions, inflammatory lung processes, brown fat uptake, second primary malignancies, radiotherapy-induced pneumonitis, and thymus hyperplasia (especially in children and young adults) [33–36]. Thymic hyperplasia is a common phenomenon that occurs after completion of treatment. It has been proposed that this finding is due to an immunologic rebound characterized by thymic aplasia followed by hyperplasia [37]. For illustrations see Figs. 2.1, 2.2, 2.3, 2.4, 2.5, 2.6, and 2.7.

In some cases, uncertainty will exist, and discussion concerning true positive PET lesions (i.e., persisting Hodgkin activity) or false-positive PET lesions (i.e., inflammation following treatment) cannot be resolved. In such clinical situations, an often invasive biopsy procedure is the only solution to bring clarity. If such a surgical intervention is not feasible, the alternative option can be to perform a PET/CT scan after 2–3 months. Recently we have treated a young man with relapsed Hodgkin lymphoma, with nodal involvement in the axillary lymph nodes, just outside the radiation field. His original disease was located in the cervical and mediastinal region. During second-line treatment with DHAP and brentuximab vedotin (clinical trial Phase II), his axillary lymph nodes disappeared, but a new lesion came up in the mediastinal area. Discussion about the origin of this new lesion could not be settled. We have asked the thoracic surgeon to perform a mediastinotomy and remove the PET-positive lesion. It appeared to be fibrotic tissue with sheets of active macrophage involvement and debris. He remained in complete remission after autologous stem cell transplantation.

2.6   Technical Considerations

Although never studied in detail, it might be expected that assessment of PET/CT for post-treatment evaluation in HL is more accurate than assessment of PET "stand-alone" imaging results. Especially for the proper evaluation of FDG uptake in the mediastinal region, a secure correlation with anatomical structures is essential.

Fig. 2.1 (**a**) A 35-year-old female with biopsy-proven Hodgkin's disease; the figure represents the initial FDG-PET/CT scan, which was used for staging. The findings are consistent with bulky mediastinal nodal Hodgkin's lymphoma. (**b**) FDG-PET/CT restaging after chemother- apy (BEACOPP escalated). The post-therapy scan shows a residual mediastinal mass on the CT images (*red arrow*). The FDG uptake was low reflecting an uptake intensity of 2 of the 5-point scale (5-PS), consistent with a complete metabolic response with a residual mass

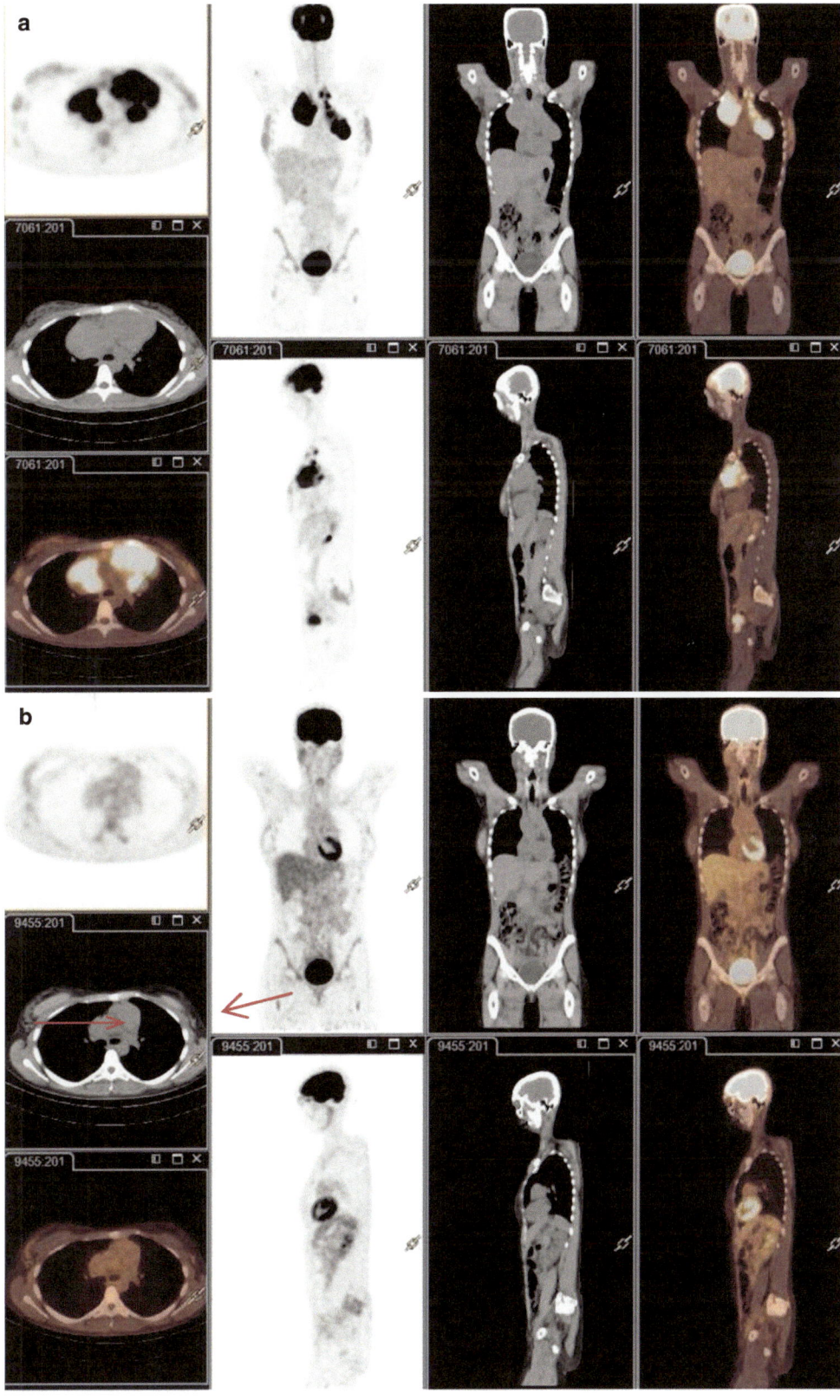

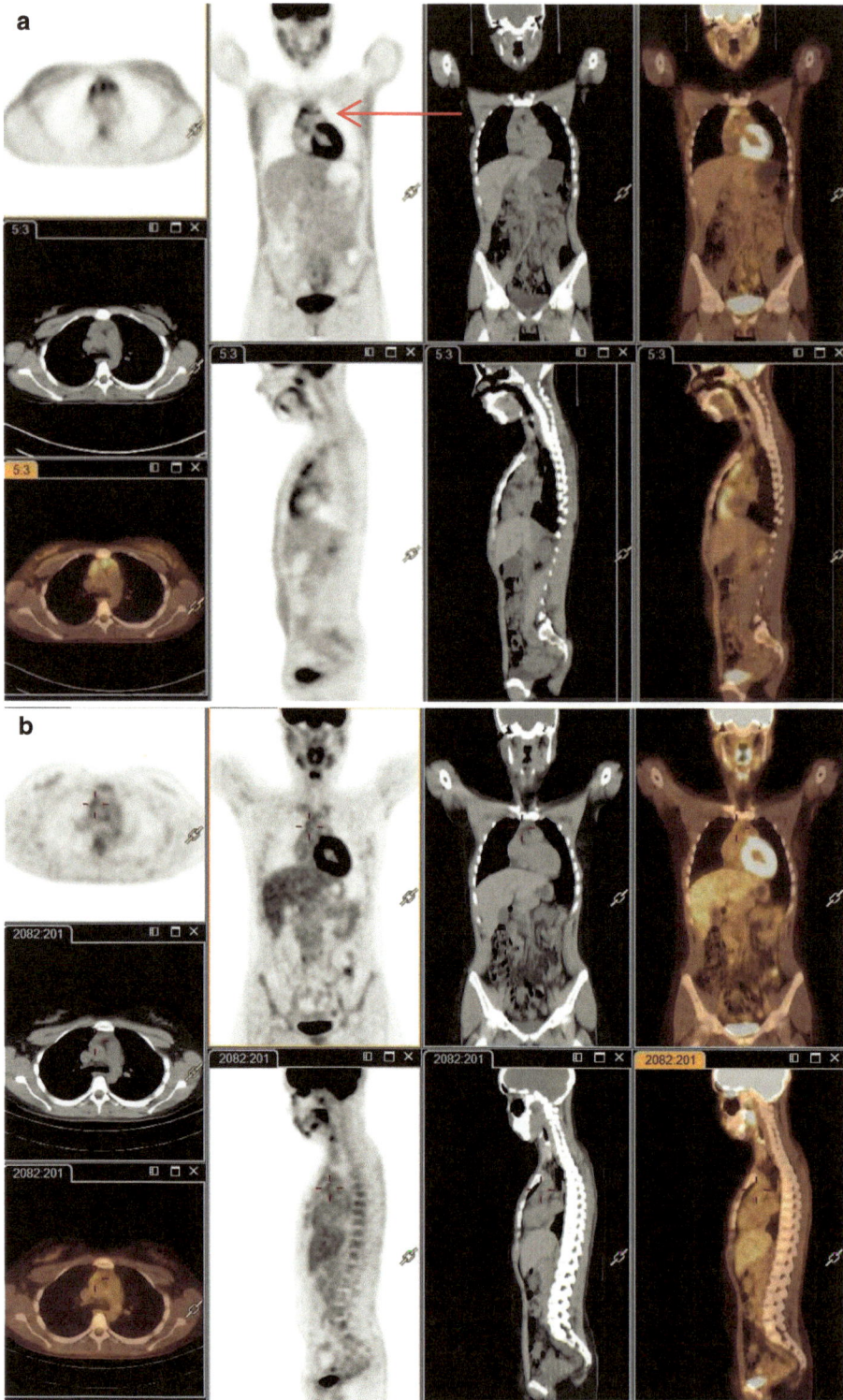

Fig. 2.2 (**a**) Follow-up FDG-PET scan in 22-year-old patient with HL, located in mediastinum and cervical lymph nodes. The posttreatment PET scan shows increased uptake in the mediastinal area (tracer uptake intensity 4 of the 5-PS); however, pattern and intensity of the FDG uptake are consistent with thymic FDG uptake in a young adoles-cent. (**b**) A PET scan performed 4 months later during follow-up demonstrated a spontaneous regression of rebound uptake in thymus. This observation was consistent with the clinical course showing no relapse of HL in this patient. *Red arrow* pointing to the mediastinal FDG uptake

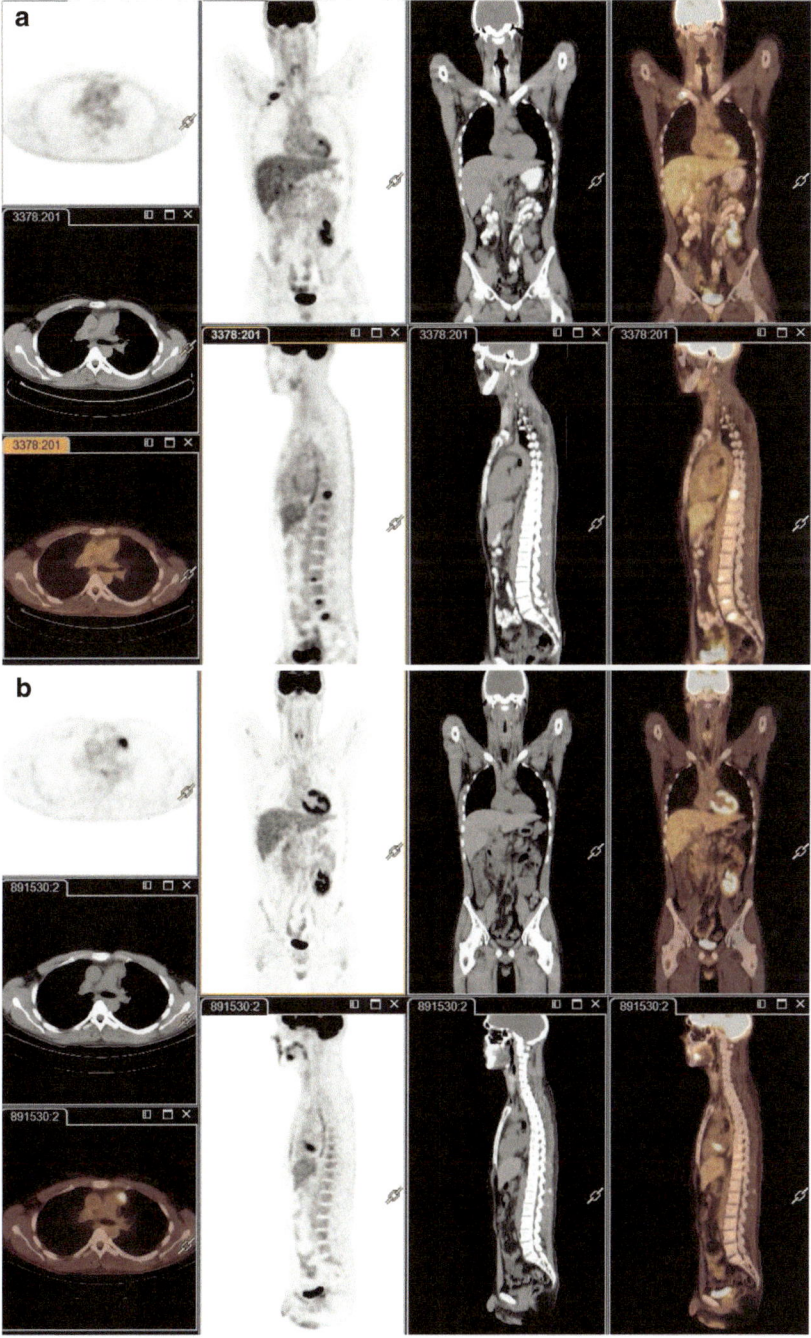

Fig. 2.3 (**a**) A 23-year-old patient with initial bulky mediastinal HL (stage IV); patient was treated with BEACOPP chemotherapy and mediastinal radiotherapy. After this initial treatment schedule, a FDG-PET scan showed a relapsed HL with nodal infraclavicular disease and extra-nodal localization in the spine. (**b**) After treatment with DHAP chemotherapy, the PET/CT scan demonstrated a good treatment response with no FDG uptake in the infraclavicular nodal region and in the extra-nodal vertebral localizations (see coronal and sagittal views). However, this PET scan showed intense uptake in the mediastinal region (transaxial PET image **b**). This nodal uptake was not visible on the pretreatment scan at relapse (see axial image **a**). Therefore, a biopsy was performed. The biopsy of the mediastinal node with increased FDG uptake revealed the presence of macrophages and lymphocytes in a lymph node. Hence, this mediastinal FDG uptake reflected a false-positive lesion with a local inflammatory response

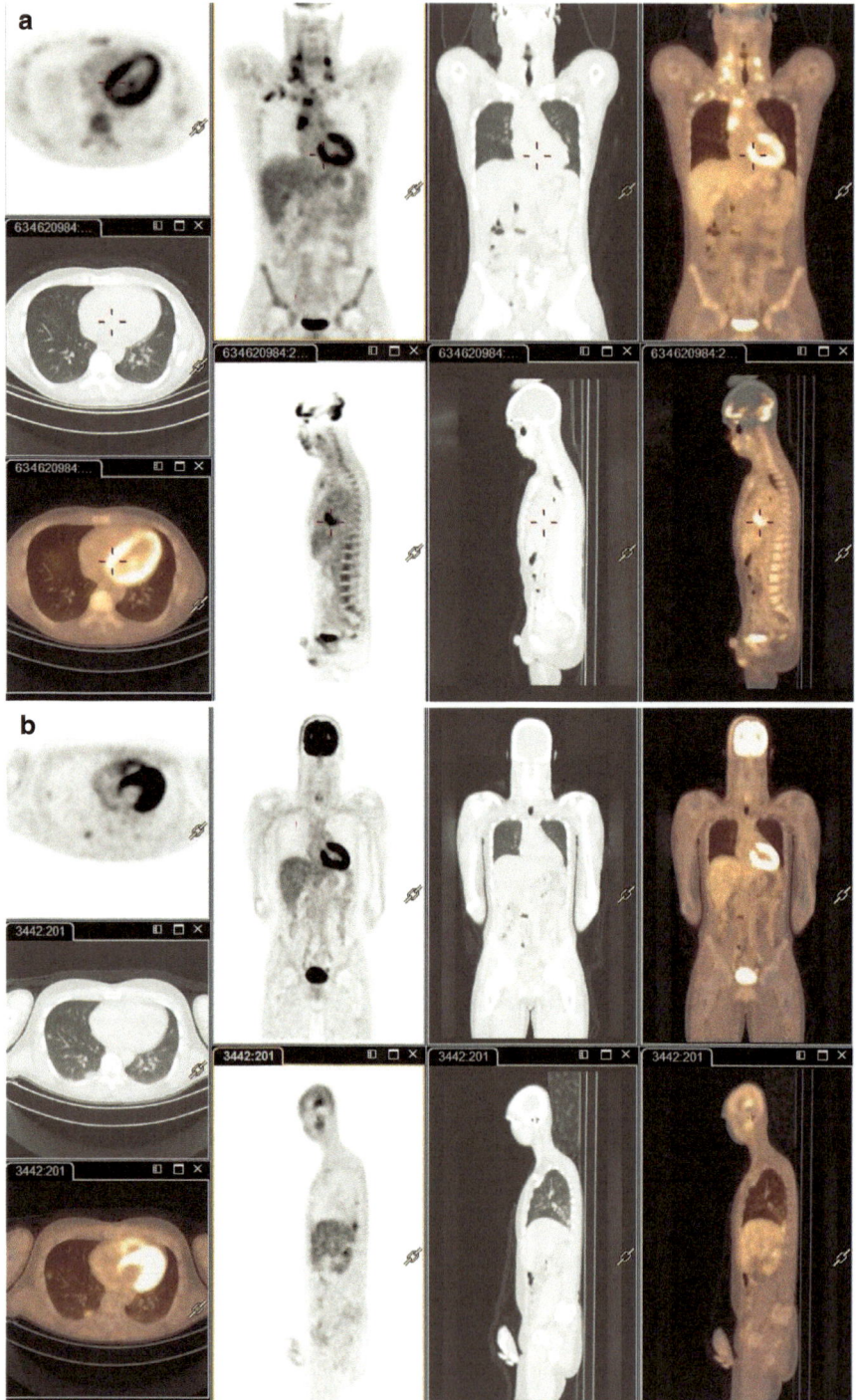

Fig. 2.4 (**a**) Baseline FDG-PET/CT in staging HL with intense FDG uptake in nodular disease in the cervical regions, mediastinum, and right axilla. (**b**) FDG-PET/CT after chemotherapy. The PET scan showed disappearance of the FDG uptake in the initial nodal localizations reflecting a complete metabolic response; however, two sites with FDG uptake were seen in the right lung (axial image). The lung uptake was new compared to the baseline PET scan (compare axial images **a** and **b**); therefore, the pulmonary lesions were classified as a category X of the 5-PS ("new areas of uptake unlikely to be related to lymphoma") representing inflammatory parenchymal lung uptake (infection)

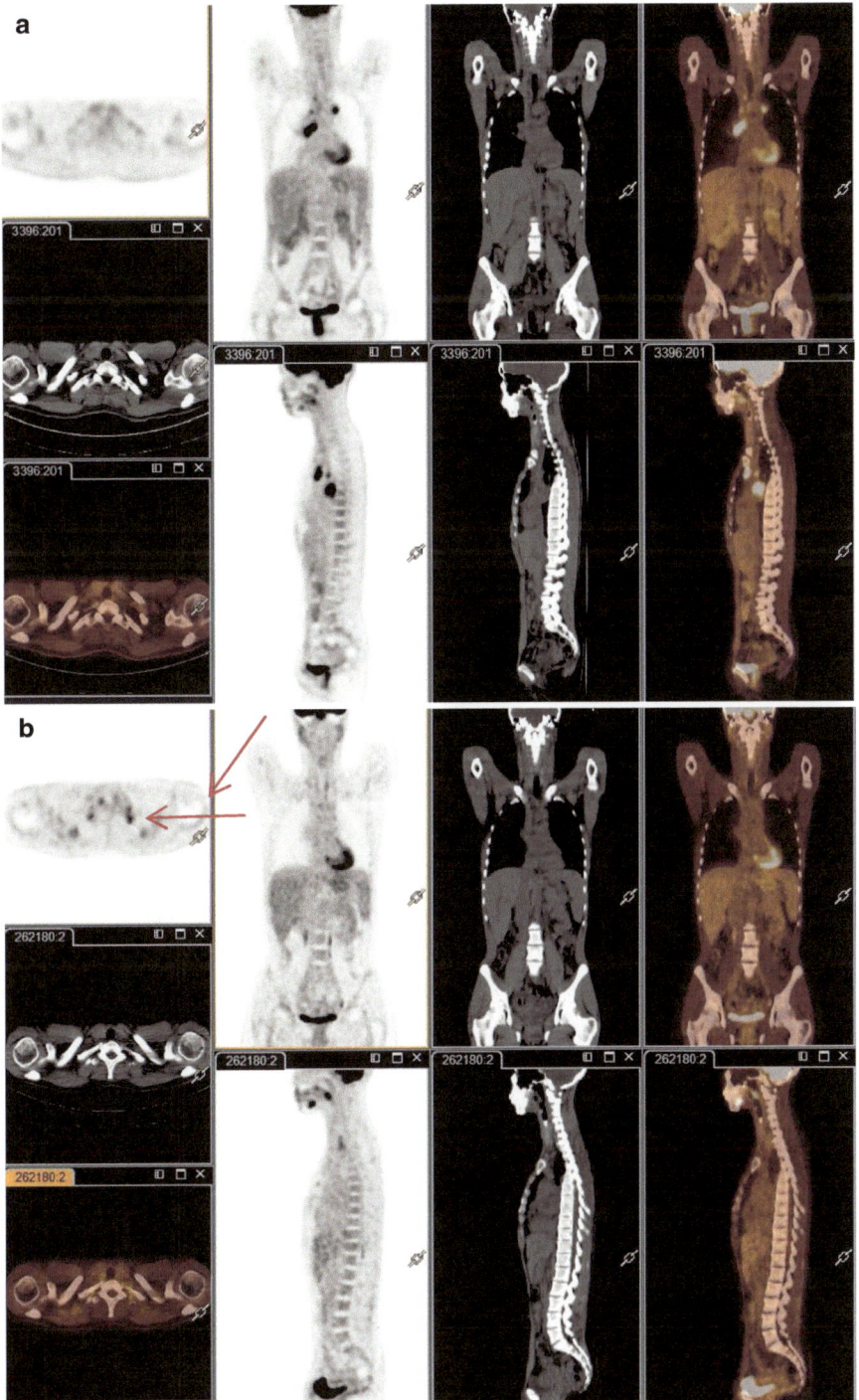

Fig. 2.5 (**a**) FDG-PET/CT staging of HL patient with nodal mediastinal disease (see coronal and sagittal images). (**b**) The posttreatment PET/CT after ABVD showed a complete metabolic response (compare coronal and sagittal images of **a** and **b**); however, symmetric cervical FDG uptake was seen (*arrow*, axial images **b**). These cervical localizations were new compared to the baseline PET scan (axial image **a**). Correlation with the CT images demonstrated no nodal FDG uptake, but FDG uptake in fat, consistent with symmetric brown fat uptake. Altogether, the cervical uptake was classified as an X classification of the 5-PS. *Red arrow* pointing to the cervical FDG uptake

Using PET/CT instead of PET and separate CT facilitates a more accurate assessment.

In the current Lugano criteria, a staging PET/CT is not only advised but mandatory for a good posttreatment evaluation [17].

2.7   Practical Considerations

For ordering physicians, it is important that they understand the clinical information needed by imaging physicians to optimize the interpretation of such studies. The request for the PET/CT examination should include sufficient medical information to demonstrate medical necessity and should at least include the diagnosis and questions to be answered. For posttreatment evaluation, it is essential that recent infections, comorbidity, and diabetes mellitus are mentioned. The results of prior imaging studies should be available to review, including planar radiography, CT, and staging FDG-PET/CT. An overview of used medication, especially antidiabetic medication, corticosteroids, and growth factors and in the case of therapy evaluation type and date of last chemotherapy or radiotherapy must be mentioned [30].

The timing for end-of-treatment evaluation PET should be at least 3 weeks after chemotherapy [8] and preferably 8–12 weeks after completion of radiotherapy. This approach should be adopted to improve diagnostic accuracy by avoiding post-therapy inflammatory changes.

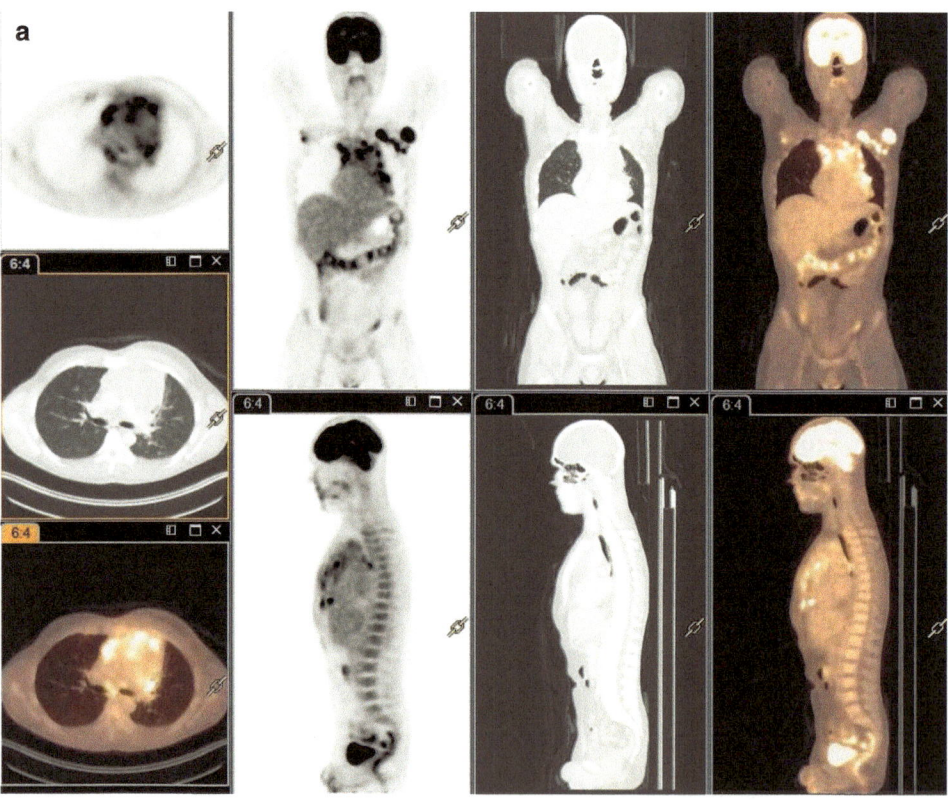

Fig. 2.6 (**a**) FDG-PET/CT scan of patient with a relapsed HL; images show intense uptake in the mediastinal and axillary lymph nodes. The FDG uptake in the bowel has a diffuse pattern and does not reflect HL. (**b**) A posttreatment FDG-PET scan showed a good treatment response. However, the PET images revealed a new focus with intense FDG uptake in the left lung (PET classification: left lung focus, category X, inflammatory FDG uptake due to pulmonal infection). (**c**) During follow-up, the pulmonary infection was treated with antibiotics, and the FDG-PET scan showed a regression of the pulmonary infection. However, this end-of-treatment PET scan showed increased uptake in the left axillary region (intensity 4 on the 5-PS), reflecting a partial remission of HL

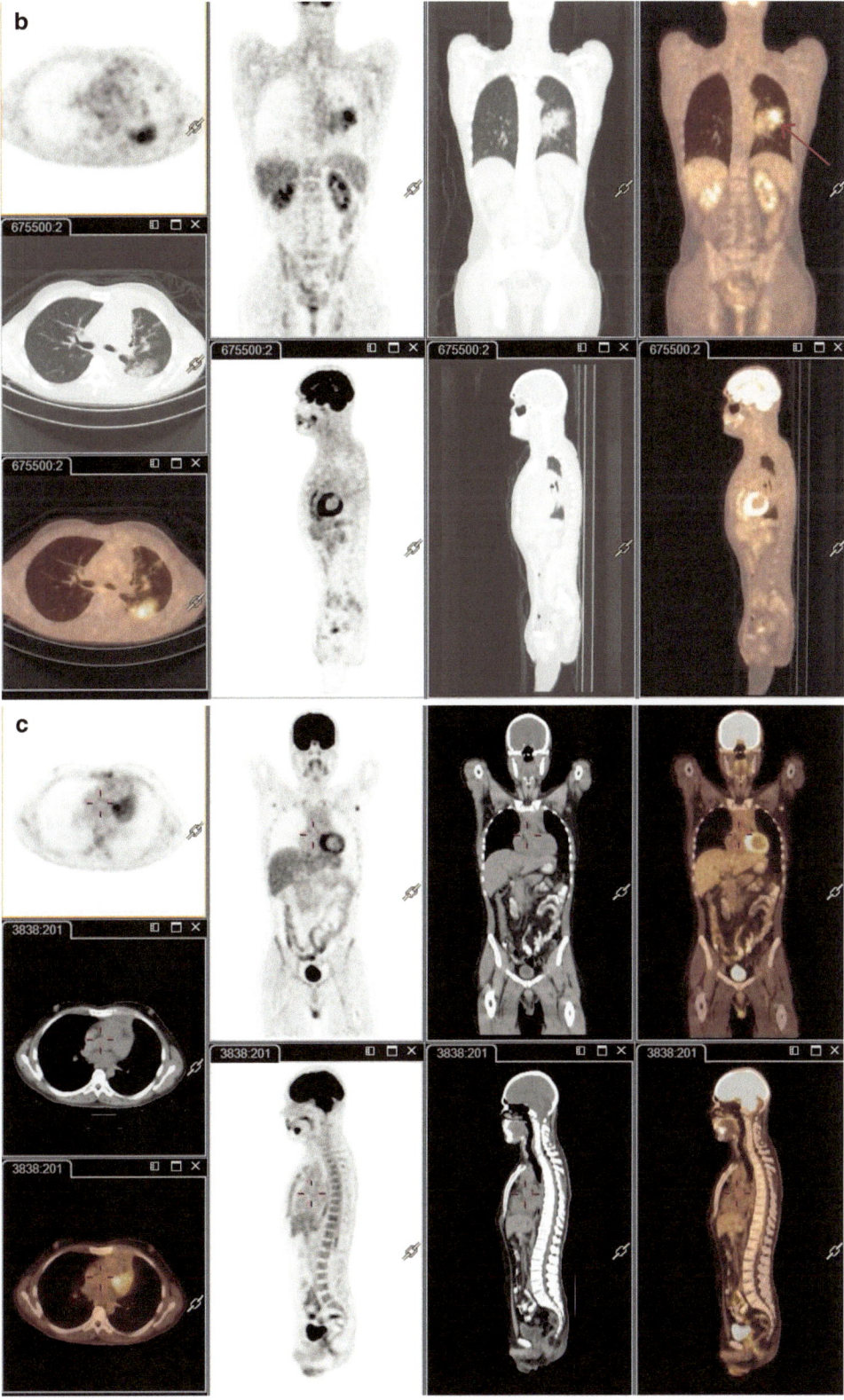

Fig. 2.6 (continued)

2.8 PET-Guided Radiotherapy as Consolidation Treatment Following Chemotherapy

By using PET/CT for response assessment after chemotherapy, the use of radiotherapy as consolidation has greatly diminished. In former days, most patients with residual tissue on CT after chemotherapy received adjuvant radiotherapy. However, with the introduction of PET/CT, it is known that even for patients with large residual masses, but without FDG avidity, there is no need for radiotherapy. The negative predictive value (NPV) of FDG-PET has been investigated by the German Hodgkin Study Group in the HD15 trial.

In this trial, patients with advanced stage HL were treated with 6 or 8 cycles of BEACOPP. The NPV appeared to be 94 % after a follow-up of 12 months. Thus, following BEACOPP consolidation radiotherapy can be omitted in PET(−) patients with residual disease without increasing the risk for progression or early relapse compared with patients in complete remission [38, 39]. In this trial, only 11 % of patients appeared to be PET(+) and received additional radiotherapy. For advanced stage HL patients treated with ABVD, PET-guided radiotherapy has not been validated. However, there are no arguments to doubt on the relevance of PET-guided radiotherapy in this setting.

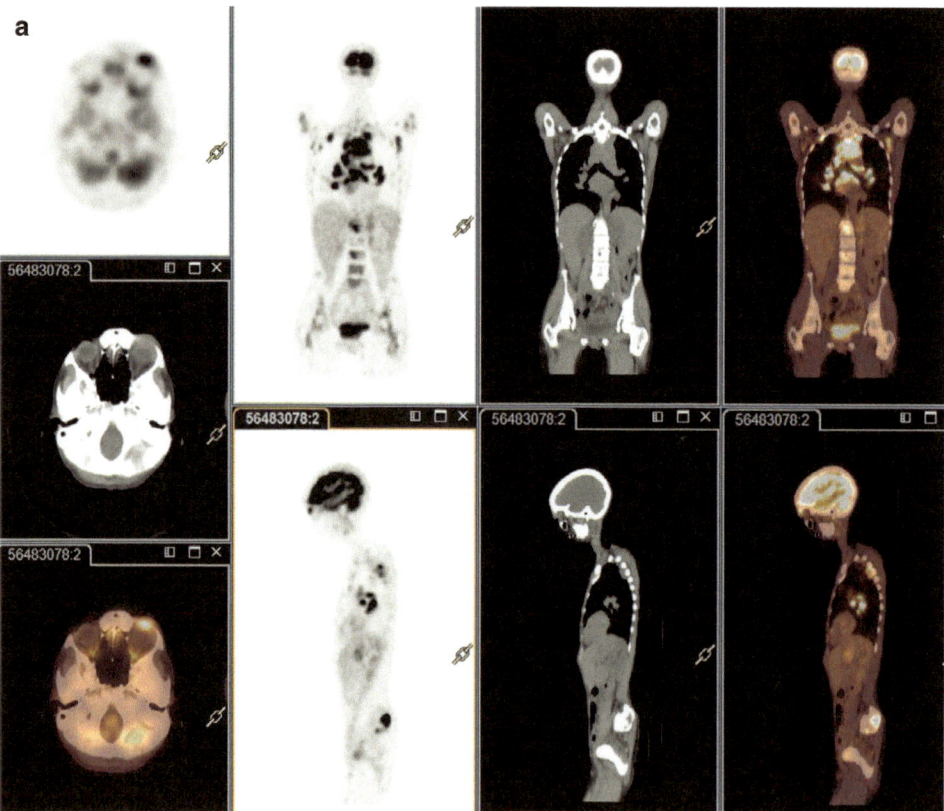

Fig. 2.7 (a) Patient with known sarcoidosis in the mediastinum and hilar lymph nodes, presented with a localization of Hodgkin lymphoma in left orbital region (rare localization, biopsy proven); see axial image. FDG-PET demonstrating intense FDG uptake in orbital region, mediastinal and hilar FDG uptake, and ossal foci. (b) Posttreatment FDG-PET showing regression of the orbital lesion and the bone marrow localizations (see axial and sagittal images). However, mediastinal and hilar FDG uptake remains abnormal with multiple focal areas with increased FDG uptake. This uptake may reflect sarcoidosis or a partial response. (c) During follow-up an additional FDG-PET scan was performed. During follow-up the biopsy-proven HL site in the orbita remained without any sign of relapse. The mediastinal and hilar FDG uptake showed some decline of FDG uptake, consistent with a decline of sarcoidosis activity. During 2 years of follow-up, no relapse of HL was observed

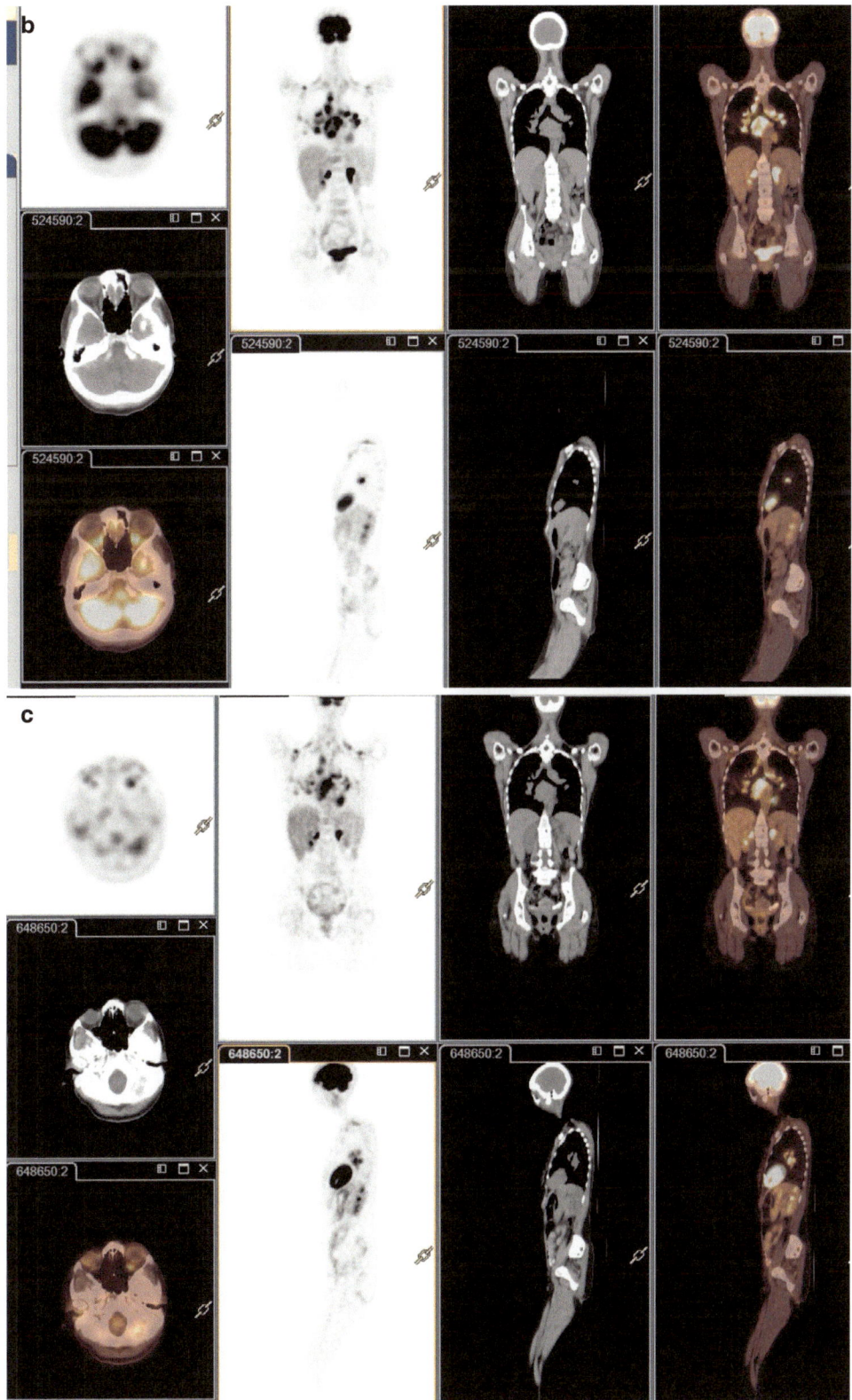

Fig. 2.7 (continued)

References

1. Cartwright RA, Watkins G. Epidemiology of Hodgkin's disease: a review. Hematol Oncol. 2004;22:11–26.

2. Hoh CK, Glaspy J, Rosen P, Dahlbom M, Lee SJ, Kunkel L, Hawkin RA, Maddahi J, Phelps ME. Whole-body FDG-PET imaging for staging of Hodgkin's disease and lymphoma. J Nucl Med. 1997;38:343–8.

3. Juweid ME, Cheson BD. Role of positron emission tomography in lymphoma. J Clin Oncol. 2005;23: 4577–80.

4. Cheson BD, Horning SJ, Coiffier B, Shipp MA, Fisher RI, Connors JM, Lister TA, Vose J, Grillo-López A, Hagenbeek A, Cabanillas F, Klippensten D, Hiddemann W, Castellino R, Harris NL, Armitage JO, Carter W, Hoppe R, Canellos GP. Report of an international workshop to standardize response criteria for non-Hodgkin's lymphomas. NCI Sponsored International Working Group. J Clin Oncol. 1999;17:1244.

5. Hoekstra OS, Ossenkoppele GJ, Golding R, van Lingen A, Visser GW, Teule GJ, Huijgens PC. Early treatment response in malignant lymphoma, as determined by planar fluorine-18-fluorodeoxyglucose scintigraphy. J Nucl Med. 1993;34:1706–10.

6. Juweid ME, Wiseman GA, Vose JM, Ritchie JM, Menda Y, Wooldridge JE, Mottaghy FM, Rohren EM, Blumstein NM, Stolpen A, Link BK, Reske SN, Graham MM, Cheson BD. Response assessment of aggressive non-Hodgkin's lymphoma by integrated International Workshop Criteria and fluorine-18-fluorodeoxyglucose positron emission tomography. J Clin Oncol. 2005;23:4652–61.

7. Cheson BD, Pfistner B, Juweid ME, Gascoyne RD, Specht L, Horning SJ, Coiffier B, Fisher RI, Hagenbeek A, Zucca E, Rosen ST, Stroobants S, Lister TA, Hoppe RT, Dreyling M, Tobinai K, Vose JM, Connors JM, Federico M, Diehl V, International Harmonization Project on Lymphoma. Revised response criteria for malignant lymphoma. J Clin Oncol. 2007;25:579–86.

8. Juweid ME, Stroobants S, Hoekstra OS, Mottaghy FM, Dietlein M, Guermazi A, Wiseman GA, Kostakoglu L, Scheidhauer K, Buck A, Naumann R, Spaepen K, Hicks RJ, Weber WA, Reske SN, Schwaiger M, Schwartz LH, Zijlstra JM, Siegel BA, Cheson BD. Imaging Subcommittee of International Harmonization Project in Lymphoma. J Clin Oncol. 2007;25:571–8.

9. Jerusalem G, Beguin Y, Fassotte MF, et al. Whole-body positron emission tomography using 18F-fluorodeoxyglucose for posttreatment evaluation in Hodgkin's disease and non-Hodgkin's lymphoma has higher diagnostic and prognostic value than classical computed tomography scan imaging. Blood. 1999;94:429–33.

10. Spaepen K, Stroobants S, Dupont P, et al. Prognostic value of positron emission tomography (PET) with fluorine-18 fluorodeoxyglucose ([18F]FDG) after first-line chemotherapy in non-Hodgkin's lymphoma: is [18F]FDG-PET a valid alternative to conventional diagnostic methods? J Clin Oncol. 2001;19:414–9.

11. de Wit M, Bohuslavizki KH, Buchert R, et al. 18FDG-PET following treatment as valid predictor for disease-free survival in Hodgkin's lymphoma. Ann Oncol. 2001;12:29–37.

12. de Wit M, Bumann D, Beyer W, et al. Whole-body positron emission tomography (PET) for diagnosis of residual mass in patients with lymphoma. Ann Oncol. 1997;8 Suppl 1:57–60.

13. Naumann R, Vaic A, Beuthien-Baumann B, et al. Prognostic value of positron emission tomography in the evaluation of post-treatment residual mass in patients with Hodgkin's disease and non-Hodgkin's lymphoma. Br J Haematol. 2001;115:793–800.

14. Weihrauch MR, Re D, Scheidhauer K, et al. Thoracic positron emission tomography using 18F-fluorodeoxyglucose for the evaluation of residual mediastinal Hodgkin disease. Blood. 2001;98:2930–4.

15. Canellos GP. Residual mass in lymphoma may not be residual disease. J Clin Oncol. 1988;6:931–3.

16. Cheson BD, Fisher RI, Barrington SF, Cavalli F, Schwartz LH, Zucca E, Lister TA, Alliance, Australasian Leukaemia and Lymphoma Group, Eastern Cooperative Oncology Group, European Mantle Cell Lymphoma Consortium, Italian Lymphoma Foundation, European Organisation for Research, Treatment of Cancer/Dutch Hemato-Oncology Group, Grupo Español de Médula Ósea, German High-Grade Lymphoma Study Group, German Hodgkin's Study Group, Japanese Lymphorra Study Group, Lymphoma Study Association, NCIC Clinical Trials Group, Nordic Lymphoma Study Group, Southwest Oncology Group, United Kingdom National Cancer Research Institute. Recommendations for initial evaluation, staging, and response assessment of Hodgkin and non-Hodgkin lymphoma: the Lugano classification. J Clin Oncol. 2014;32: 3059–68.

17. Barrington SF, Mikhaeel NG, Kostakoglu L, Meignan M, Hutchings M, Müeller SP, Schwartz LH, Zucca E, Fisher RI, Trotman J, Hoekstra OS, Hicks RJ, O'Doherty MJ, Hustinx R, Biggi A, Cheson BD. Role of imaging in the staging and response assessment of lymphoma: consensus of the International Conference on Malignant Lymphomas Imaging Working Group. J Clin Oncol. 2014;32:3048–58.

18. Zijlstra JM, Lindauer-van der Werf G, Hoekstra OS, Hooft L, Riphagen II, Huijgens PC. 18F-fluorodeoxyglucose positron emission tomography for posttreatment evaluation of malignant lymphoma: a systematic review. Haematologica. 2006;91:522–9.

19. Terasawa T, Nihashi T, Hotta T, Nagai H. 18F-FDG PET for posttherapy assessment of Hodgkin's disease and aggressive Non-Hodgkin's lymphoma: a systematic review. J Nucl Med. 2008;49:13–21.

20. Morbelli S, Capitanio S, De Carli F, Bongioanni F, De Astis E, Miglino M, Verardi MT, Buschiazzo A, Fiz F,

Marini C, Pomposelli E, Sambuceti G. Baseline and ongoing PET-derived factors predict detrimental effect or potential utility of 18F-FDG PET/CT (FDG-PET/CT) performed for surveillance in asymptomatic lymphoma patients in first remission. Eur J Nucl Med Mol Imaging. 2016;43(2):232–9.

21. Juweid ME. FDG-PET/CT in lymphoma. Methods Mol Biol. 2011;727:1–19. doi:10.1007/978-1-61779-062-1_1.

22. Kobe C, Kuhnert G, Kahraman D, Haverkamp H, Eich HT, Franke M, Persigehl T, Klutmann S, Amthauer H, Bockisch A, Kluge R, Wolf HH, Maintz D, Fuchs M, Borchmann P, Diehl V, Drzezga A, Engert A, Dietlein M. Assessment of tumor size reduction improves outcome prediction of positron emission tomography/computed tomography after chemotherapy in advanced-stage Hodgkin lymphoma. J Clin Oncol. 2014;32:1776–81.

23. Gerrie AS, Power MM, Shepherd JD, Savage KJ, Sehn LH, Connors JM. Chemoresistance can be overcome with high-dose chemotherapy and autologous stem-cell transplantation for relapsed and refractory Hodgkin lymphoma. Ann Oncol. 2014;25:2218–23.

24. Rancea M, von Tresckow B, Monsef I, Engert A, Skoetz N. High-dose chemotherapy followed by autologous stem cell transplantation for patients with relapsed or refractory Hodgkin lymphoma: a systematic review with meta-analysis. Crit Rev Oncol Hematol. 2014;92:1–10.

25. Gentzler RD, Evens AM, Rademaker AW, Weitner BB, Mittal BB, Dillehay GL, Petrich AM, Altman JK, Frankfurt O, Variakojis D, Singhal S, Mehta J, Williams S, Kaminer L, Gordon LI, Winter JN. F-18 FDG-PET predicts outcomes for patients receiving total lymphoid irradiation and autologous blood stem-cell transplantation for relapsed and refractory Hodgkin lymphoma. Br J Haematol. 2014;165:793–800.

26. Devillier R, Coso D, Castagna L, Brenot Rossi I, Anastasia A, Chiti A, Ivanov V, Schiano JM, Santoro A, Chabannon C, Balzarotti M, Blaise D, Bouabdallah R. Positron emission tomography response at the time of autologous stem cell transplantation predicts outcome of patients with relapsed and/or refractory Hodgkin's lymphoma responding to prior salvage therapy. Haematologica. 2012;97:1073–9.

27. Moskowitz CH, Matasar MJ, Zelenetz AD, Nimer SD, Gerecitano J, Hamlin P, Horwitz S, Moskowitz AJ, Noy A, Palomba L, Perales MA, Portlock C, Straus D, Maragulia JC, Schoder H, Yahalom J. Normalization of pre-ASCT, FDG-PET imaging with second-line, non-cross-resistant, chemotherapy programs improves event-free survival in patients with Hodgkin lymphoma. Blood. 2012;119:1665–70.

28. Poulou LS, Thanos L, Ziakas PD. Unifying the predictive value of pretransplant FDG PET in patients with lymphoma: a review and meta-analysis of published trials. Eur J Nucl Med Mol Imaging. 2010;37:156–62.

29. Martelli M, Ceriani L, Zucca E, Zinzani PL, Ferreri AJ, Vitolo U, Stelitano C, Brusamolino E, Cabras MG, Rigacci L, Balzarotti M, Salvi F, Montoto S, Lopez-Guillermo A, Finolezzi E, Pileri SA, Davies A, Cavalli F, Giovanella L, Johnson PW. [18F]fluorodeoxyglucose positron emission tomography predicts survival after chemoimmunotherapy for primary mediastinal large B-cell lymphoma: results of the International Extranodal Lymphoma Study Group IELSG-26 Study. J Clin Oncol. 2014;32:1769–75.

30. Boellaard R, Delgado-Bolton R, Oyen WJ, Giammarile F, Tatsch K, Eschner W, Verzijlbergen FJ, Barrington SF, Pike LC, Weber WA, Stroobants S, Delbeke D, Donohoe KJ, Holbrook S, Graham MM, Testanera G, Hoekstra OS, Zijlstra J, Visser E, Hoekstra CJ, Pruim J, Willemsen A, Arends B, Kotzerke J, Bockisch A, Beyer T, Chiti A, Krause BJ. FDG PET/CT: EANM procedure guidelines for tumour imaging: version 2.0. Eur J Nucl Med Mol Imaging. 2015;42(2):328–54.

31. Paes FM, Kalkanis DG, Sideras PA, Serafini AN. FDG PET/CT of extranodal involvement in non-Hodgkin lymphoma and Hodgkin disease. Radiographics. 2010;30:269–91.

32. Hunt BM, Vallières E, Buduhan G, Aye R, Louie B. Sarcoidosis as a benign cause of lymphadenopathy in cancer patients. Am J Surg. 2009;197:629–32.

33. Biggi A, Gallamini A, Chauvie S, Hutchings M, Kostakoglu L, Gregianin M, Meignan M, Malkowski B, Hofman MS, Barrington SF. International validation study for interim PET in ABVD-treated, advanced-stage hodgkin lymphoma: interpretation criteria and concordance rate among reviewers. J Nucl Med. 2013;54:683–90.

34. Molnar Z, Simon Z, Borbenyi Z, Deak B, Galuska L, Keresztes K, Miltenyi Z, Marton I, Rosta A, Schneider T, Tron L, Varady E, Illes A. Prognostic value of FDG-PET in Hodgkin lymphoma for posttreatment evaluation. Long term follow-up results. Neoplasma. 2010;57:349–54.

35. Quarles van Ufford H, Hoekstra O, de Haas M, Fijnheer R, Wittebol S, Tieks B, Kramer M, de Klerk J. On the added value of baseline FDG-PET in malignant lymphoma. Mol Imaging Biol. 2010;12:225–32.

36. Schöder H, Moskowitz C. PET imaging for response assessment in lymphoma: potential and limitations. Radiol Clin North Am. 2008;46:225–41.

37. Fallanca F, Giovacchini G, Ponzoni M, Gianolli L, Ciceri F, Fazio F. Cervical thymic hyperplasia after chemotherapy in an adult patient with Hodgkin lymphoma: a potential cause of false-positivity on [18F] FDG PET/CT scanning. Br J Haematol. 2008;140:477.

38. Kobe C, Dietlein M, Franklin J, Markova J, Lohri A, Amthauer H, Klutmann S, Knapp WH, Zijlstra JM, Bockisch A, Weckesser M, Lorenz R, Schreckenberger M, Bares R, Eich HT, Mueller RP, Fuchs M, Borchmann P, Schicha H, Diehl V, Engert A. Positron emission tomography has a high negative predictive value for progression or early relapse for patients with residual disease after first-line chemotherapy in advanced-stage Hodgkin lymphoma. Blood. 2008; 112:3989–94.

39. Engert A, Haverkamp H, Kobe C, Markova J, Renner C, Ho A, Zijlstra J, Král Z, Fuchs M, Hallek M,

Kanz L, Döhner H, Dörken B, Engel N, Topp M, Klutmann S, Amthauer H, Bockisch A, Kluge R, Kratochwil C, Schober O, Greil R, Andreesen R, Kneba M, Pfreundschuh M, Stein H, Eich HT, Müller RP, Dietlein M, Borchmann P, Diehl V. Reduced-intensity chemotherapy and PET-guided radiotherapy in patients with advanced stage Hodgkin's lymphoma (HD15 trial): a randomised, open-label, phase 3 non-inferiority trial. Lancet. 2012;379:1791–9.

40. Juweid ME. 18F-FDG PET as a routine test for post-therapy assessment of Hodgkin's disease and aggressive non-Hodgkin's lymphoma: where is the evidence? J Nucl Med. 2008;49:9–12.

Andrea Gallamini, Anna Borra,
and Colette Zwarthoed

3.1   Introduction

Since chemotherapy inception in the early 1950s, the prediction of the ultimate treatment response has been the object of intensive clinical research in oncology for more than half a century. In the millennium turnaround, this interest has been further fuelled by the technological progress of medical imaging for cancer treatment monitoring and by the discovery of a vast array of new prognostic and predictive markers for a modern, personalized treatment strategy. The concept of prognostication does not necessarily overlap with treatment response prediction. In general, prognostic markers are readily available before treatment onset, are informative of the risk of recurrence, and on the ultimate treatment outcome of a given malignancy. They are useful to minimize confounding factors when comparing the results of similar cohorts of patients in clinical trials, or when stratifying patients according to their risk of treatment failure. On the other hand, predictive markers are treatment-dependent and available only during therapy. Tumour response prediction, based on the early appraisal of a number of tumour biomarkers, which proved informative of the final treatment outcome, is increasingly used in Oncology [1]. Tumour chemosensitivity was originally studied from in vitro cultures of cancer cells from patient, and has been considered for long the ideal predictive tool of final treatment outcome [2]. Standard parameters such as colony-forming ability, growth inhibition, or cell viability were used as measurable indexes of sensitivity to cytostatic drugs. Later on, the development of high-throughput technologies, e.g. cDNA microarrays, enabled a more detailed analysis of drug responses. However, these methods proved unsuitable in the clinical practice and they are currently limited to new drug discovery and preclinical drug testing platforms [3]. Tumour shrinkage has been also considered in the past a surrogate marker for chemosensitivity, and classical radiological imaging by contrast-enhanced computed tomography (CeCT) scan has been proposed during treatment to assess an early tumour response [4]. However, it became clear that traditional radiological assessment of tumour bulk shrinkage is not an accurate

Prof. A. Gallamini (✉)
Research, Innovation and Statistics Department,
A. Lacassagne Cancer Centre,
33, Rue de Valombrose, Nice 06189, France
e-mail: andreagallamini@gmail.com,
andrea.GALLAMINI@nice.unicancer.fr

A. Borra
Hematology and Bone Marrow Transplant
Department, Azienda Ospedaliera S. Croce e Carle,
Cuneo, Italy

C. Zwarthoed
Nuclear Medicine Department, A. Lacassagne Cancer
Centre, Nice, France

© Springer International Publishing Switzerland 2016   31
A. Gallamini (ed.), *PET Scan in Hodgkin Lymphoma*, DOI 10.1007/978-3-319-31797-7_3

predictor of outcome, as any reduction in tumour volume takes time and can lag behind metabolic slowdown of the neoplastic tissue, which occurs immediately after chemotherapy delivery. This is particularly evident in HL, where a residual mass is observed in up to two-thirds of the patients at the end of treatment [5, 6]. Furthermore, treatment response assessment by radiological imaging modalities may be inaccurate because of errors in tumour measurements, errors in selection of measurable targets, and inter-observer variability of tumor size assessment [7]. More recently, a new class of prgnostic markes able to predict treatment outcome in a single patients-basis have beeen proposed. Among them, functional imaging by ^{67}Ga-citrate scintigraphy or ^{18}F-fluorodeoxyglucose (FDG) positron emission tomography (FDG PET) proved able to predict treatment outcome, as surrogate markers of chemosensitivity with superior overall accuracy in lymphoma [8, 9] and other solid neoplasms [10–12]. Similarly, minimal residual disease (MRD) detection by flow cytometry or molecular biology in acute and chronic leukaemia proved essential to predict long-term disease control [13–16]. The predicted benefit (overall survival) and/or its surrogate (progression-free survival) must be appropriate to the treatment context. In this aspect a "predictive" marker is different from a "prognostic" marker since only the former is strictly related to a given treatment. In HL, this concept applies both to end of therapy and interim PET scan, whose predictive role on treatment outcome, whatever the time point during chemotherapy or chemoradiation the scan is performed, depends on the intensity of delivered therapy [17].

3.2 Interim PET to Predict Treatment Outcome

3.2.1 Prognostication in HL

HL has been for long considered the archetype in oncology for tumour staging, restaging, and prognostication. The Ann Arbor staging system [18], and later the Cotswolds revised classification [19], first introduced the concept that disease manifestations and tumour bulk identify distinct categories of patients who have a different prognosis and perhaps need specific therapeutic approaches. Surgical procedures (the so-called staging laparotomy with splenectomy and multiple nodal and organ biopsies) were first proposed in the early 1970s for tumour staging [20]. These procedures had the merit of having fuelled the knowledge on the physiopathology of disease spread, but proved cumbersome and even burdened by some morbidity. For these reasons at the beginning of the 1980s, radiological imaging with lymphography and CeCT surmounted staging laparotomy. CeCT, in particular, proved a readily accessible, non-invasive diagnostic tool, with a high sensitivity and overall accuracy for tumour spread detection and it became rapidly the standard for tumour staging [21].

In the meanwhile, the growing evidence that the tumour per se and the host reaction against the tumour were the main prognostic parameters correlated to tumour survival provided the frame for a new classification of prognostic factors in HL as (1) tumour-related, (2) host-related, and (3) environment-related [22]. Tumour-related factors include those depending on tumour biology, pathology, and burden. Host-related factors include a number of causes, which may significantly influence outcome such as age, co-morbidity, viral infections, and naïve immunity against the tumour. Environment-related factors include mainly situations outside the patients such as socio-economic status and access to god-quality health care. Assumedly, "true" prognostic factors have a known value at disease onset, before treatment starts, the so-called fixed-covariates, while others may only be known later during treatment, the so-called predictive factors or time-dependent covariates, such as time to response or early chemosensitivity assessment. The latter may be important for answering biological and clinical questions, but its prognostic relevance can be assessed only in prospective randomized studies comparing the chemosensitivity-adapted treatment (experimental arm) to the traditional non-adapted chemotherapy (standard arm) [23]. In Hl, tumour bulk, computed with a software by measuring the area of every neoplastic lesion, manually contoured in transaxial slices of CT scan by an expert radiologist, proved indeed to be one of the most powerful predictor of treatment outcome and, though related to many clinical staging parameters, was not predicted by them [24]. As a matter of fact, both in early-stage [25, 26] and in advanced-stage [27] HL, the number of involved lymph node regions as well as the volume of the disease on individual regions proved to predict progression-free survival (PFS) and overall survival (OS). These observations prompted clinicians to refine the classical four-stage Ann Arbor classification. As a consequence, a further prognostic breakdown of early-stage disease in two distinct subsets was proposed, based on a mixture of prognostic factors related to tumour bulk and host characteristics (see Table 3.1), and the intensity and duration of treatment modulated accordingly [28]. At the end of millennium, prognostic information of several biomarkers related to tumour burden and host reaction in advanced-stage disease was retrospectively extracted by a

large data set collected from 5141 advanced-stage patients treated with doxorubicin-containing regimens in 25 international institutions [29]. Seven parameters were found to be associated in multivariate analysis, with an inferior treatment outcome: low albumin levels, anaemia, male sex, age ≥ 45 year, stage IV, leucocytosis, and lymphopenia. A prognostic model, the International Prognostic Score (IPS), was then constructed, and six risk classes, depending on the number of adverse prognostic factors, were identified, showing a 5-year freedom from progression (FFP) ranging from 84 % for score 0 (no risk factor) to 42 % for score 5 (≥ 5 risk factors) (Fig. 3.1).

However, the discriminative power and the prognostic relevance of the model were limited as only 7 % of the patients showed a 6-y FFS less than 50 %, and therefore its use in clinical practice has been questioned [30]. Interestingly, nearly 20 years after, the prognostic value of IPS has been again retrospectively assessed in a comparable cohort of 686 advanced-stage HL

Table 3.1 Preliminary results of the multicentre international PET response-adapted prospective trials of the GITIL/FIL (HD0607), of the NCRI (RAPID), and of the SWOG-CALG-B (S0816)

Trial	Stage	N^a	PET-2 key	PET-2+ (%)	PET-2− (%)	3-y PFS all pts.	3-y PFS PET-2− pts.	3-y PFS PET-2+ pts.
GITIL/FIL HD 0607	IIB-IVB	656	DS	17	82	83 %	89 %[b]	66 %[b]
NCRI RATHL	IIB-IVB*	1136	DS	16	84	82 %	84–85 %[a]	68 %
SWOG S0816	III-IV	371	DS	18	82			

[a]PET-2-negative patients were randomized to ABVD vs. AVD
[b]The results in the PET-2+ and PET-2− arms are reported as 2-y PFS
*Stage II unfavourable, stage III and IV

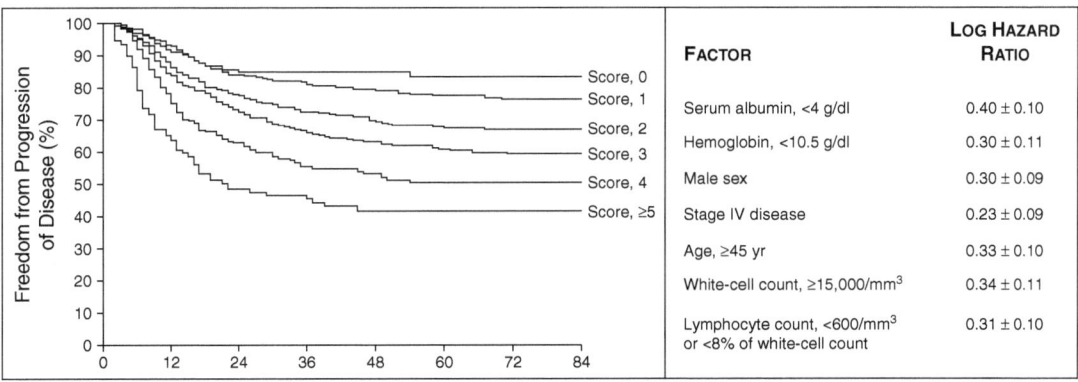

Fig. 3.1 The International Prognostic Score (IPS) for advanced-stage Hodgkin lymphoma (From Hasenclever et al. [29])

patients aged 15–65 years and staged without the contribute of FDG PET, on behalf of the British Columbia Cancer Agency (BCCA) [31]. Although confirming the prognostic role of IPS, the study showed a substantial narrowing of the distance among the 5-y FFP Kaplan-Meyer curves of the different score levels ranging between 88 % for score 0 and 70 % for score 6, that was attributed by the authors to a lower percentage of stage IV (24 % in the BCCA series vs. 42 % in the original IPS study). This phenomenon, in turn, depended on a more restrictive definition of stage IV according to BCCA guidelines. It should be stressed, however, that in the original IPS study stage IV had an adverse prognostic meaning only in the presence of 2 or more ENS attained by disease, which occurred only in 12 % of the patients. This scenario has been profoundly modified in the PET era, due to its higher sensitivity and overall accuracy comparing to CeCT in detecting ENS spread, with a resulting upward-stage migration in 20–25 % of the patients, mainly for a shift from stage III to stage IV [32].

Besides staging, HL prognostication has been also revolutionized, in the mid 1990s, by the advent of functional imaging with ^{18}F-FDG PET. In all the key aspects of HL management such as staging and restaging, early and final treatment response monitoring, radiotherapy planning, and guiding FDG PET/CT has gained an irreplaceable role, thus becoming an indissoluble and essential tool in the HL therapeutic strategy [33] (Fig. 3.2).

Probably the most relevant contribution of PET in the overall HL management has been the early chemosensitivity assessment both in early- and advanced-stage HL. This success was due to a number of tumour-related and tumour-unrelated reasons, but probably more importantly, to the peculiar pathobiology and tissue architecture of HL. The latter is characterized by the presence of few, scattered neoplastic cells, the Hodgkin and Reed-Sternberg cells (HRSC), accounting for less than 5 % of the total cell burden, embedded in a meshwork of non-neoplastic, reactive cells, which are attracted in the neoplastic milieu by a cytokine gradient and in turn responsible for the growth and immortalization of HRSCs [34]. These "inflammatory" cells, lymphocytes, macrophages, granulocytes, and eosinophils, identified as micro-environment

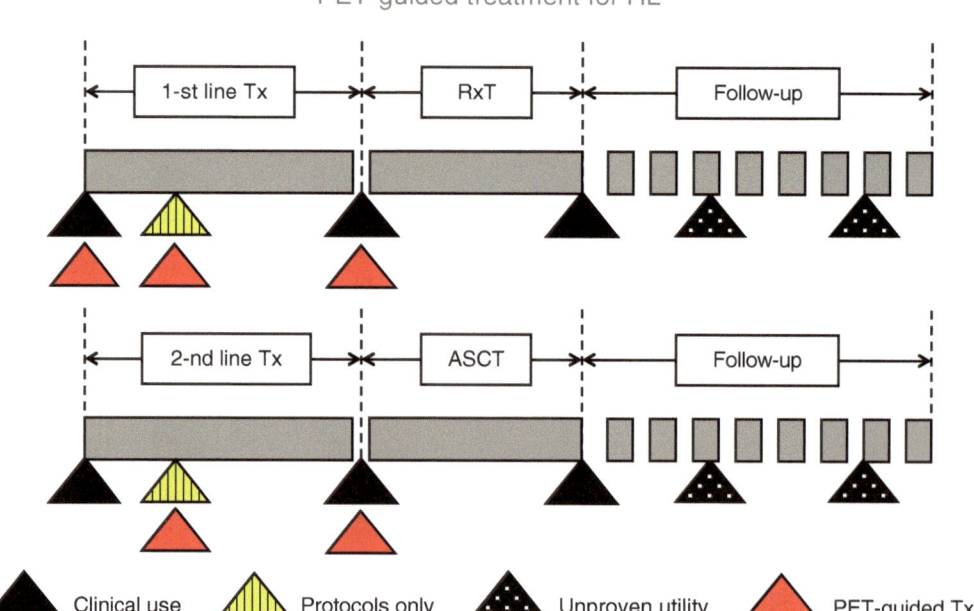

Fig. 3.2 FDG PET/CT for Hodgkin lymphoma management (Adapted from Gallamini et al. [33])

(ME) cells, show a considerably high glycolytic activity [35] and are largely responsible for the high FDG uptake within the tumour tissue [36]. Both chemokine production and metabolic activity of the ME cells are apparently shut down early during treatment in chemo-sensitive disease, in nearly in 80 % of HL patients [37–40]. In this "on-off" phenomenon, ME cells work as a signal amplifier as they are switched off in case of HRSC kill in chemo-sensitive HL and vice versa in chemo-resistant disease. This mechanism, in turn, increases dramatically the detection power of FDG PET/CT, which is normally able to detect only nodal lesion of a diameter of 4–5 mm or more [41]. As a matter of fact, interim PET scan performed after few chemotherapy courses (PET-2) with doxorubicin, bleomycin, vinblastine and dacarbazine (ABVD) is able to predict the long-term disease control with an overall high accuracy in HL, while specificity and positive predictive value (PPV) resulted higher in advanced- compared to early-stage disease [42, 43]. On the other hand, the negative predictive value (NPV) of PET-2 was reportedly very high, ranging from 100 % to 86 %, depending on the effectiveness of chemotherapy regimen [37, 44]. As mentioned above, the PPV resulted disappointingly low in early stage disease, ranging from 20 % to 45 %, probably due to (1) the high rescue rate of radiotherapy in PET-2-positive patients, (2) to the low a priori risk of treatment relapse in early-stage disease, (3) to a non-negligible rate of false-positive results due to unspecific FDG uptake in post-chemotherapy inflammatory tissue and (4) to the lack of accurate rules for interim PET reporting [42].

The situation is completely different in advanced-stage disease. In a large meta-analysis review, interim PET performed after 2 cycles of ABVD (PET-2) had an overall sensitivity of 0.81 (95 % CI, 0.72–0.89) and a specificity of 0.97 (95 % CI, 0.94–0.99) in predicting PFS [45]. In the retrospective Italian Danish study in a large ($N=260$) cohort of advanced-stage ($N=193$) or unfavourable early stage ($N=67$), treated with 6 courses of ABVD±consolidation RT, undergoing interim PET scan after 2 ABVD courses for

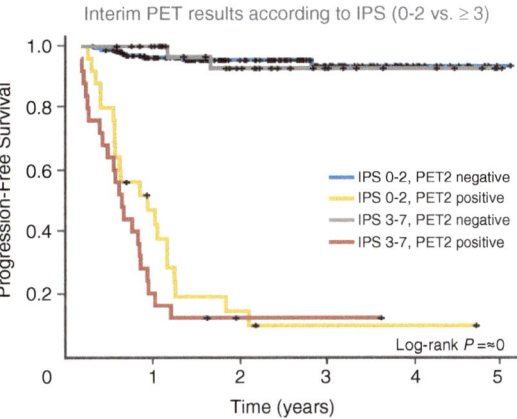

Fig. 3.3 IPS score and Interim PET scan in predicting treatment outcome in advanced-stage, ABVD-treated HL (From Gallamini et al. [8])

prognostic aim only, the 3-y PFS of PET-2-negative and PET-2-positive patients was 95 % and 12.8 % ($p<.0001$). Importantly, compared to a classical prognostic model such IPS, the predictive value of PET-2 on treatment outcome was maintained both in low- (0–2) or high-score (≥3) IPS patients, thus superseding the prognostic role of the latter [8] (Fig. 3.3).

These data have been subsequently confirmed in larger cohorts of patients [46–48]. Other groups have explored the predictive value of interim PET as early as after 1 single course of chemotherapy (PET-1). After the preliminary report in small and mixed cohort of HL and aggressive B-cell lymphoma patients, which stressed the very high negative predictive value of PET-1 [49, 50], the results of a large international prospective cooperative study have been reported in a series of 126 HL patients with early ($N=68$: 54 %) and advanced ($N=58$) stage [51]. This study confirmed the very high NPV of PET-1 of 96.8 %, while the PPV was only 44.4 %. The authors commented that if in a PET-adapted strategy the intention is treatment de-escalation – which can be an attractive option for early-stage patients – PET-1 is better than PET-2. However, because of the higher rate of false-positive results associated with PET-1, PET-2 should remain the preferred choice for selecting non responding patients to switch to a more aggressive treatment.

3.3 PET Response-Adapted Therapy

HL is a high curable disease, as most patients become long-term survivors, with a 10-year cure and survival rates after first-line treatment exceeding 80 % and 90 %, respectively [52]. However, 10–15 % of early-stage and 20–30 % of advanced-stage patients are chemo-refractory to first-line treatment, either for primary resistant or relapsing disease, and nearly half of them ultimately succumb to their disease [53]. Hence, a still unmet need exists for a valid tool to predict the completeness of therapy response and the final patient outcome. However, the most compelling argument for a personalized treatment approach based on the actual risk of chemo-resistance remains the unwarranted treatment-related morbidity. In early-stage HL, for instance, during the late follow-up, five years or more beyond diagnosis, the disease itself no longer represents the main cause of death, but secondary neoplasms and cardiovascular events do [54]. By contrast, in advanced-stage HL, the most frequent cause of death is HL (see Fig. 3.4).

However, in female aged less or more than 30 years and treated with the very active escalated BEACOPP (EB: dose-intense combination of bleomycin, etoposide, doxorubicin, cyclophosphamide, vincristine, procarbazine, and prednisolone), amenorrhoea was observed in 51 % and 95 % of the cases, respectively [55], while the cumulative risk of secondary acute myeloid leukaemia in the entire cohort of advanced-stage disease was 3 % at 10 years [56]. For these reasons the search of reliable markers for tumour response prediction in an individual basis is very attractive in the context of a highly curable neoplasm, especially in early-stage disease, in whom the rate and magnitude of treatment-related morbidity or mortality could even supersede the rate of disease-related death.

As previously mentioned, a novel class of prognostic factor in lymphoma has been proposed, based on the early individual risk assessment of chemo-resistance during treatment, either by the evaluation of MRD [57, 58] or by assessing the chemosensitivity to treatment with PET scanning. However, the clinical relevance of a prognostic factor should be weighted against its usefulness in therapy planning and effectiveness in improving overall patient treatment outcome or reducing therapy-related toxic effects without compromising treatment efficacy. Till now, nobody knows, in the absence of published results of multicentre randomized prospective trials, whether a PET-adapted strategy could ultimately improve the final outcome of high-risk HL patients or reduce toxicity in low-risk patients while maintaining the same treatment efficacy [59, 60]. Several ongoing, or already concluded prospective trials have been launched in low-risk, early- and advanced-stage HL to explore the feasibility of treatment de-escalation strategies in patients with a negative interim PET, while others have been proposed based on therapy

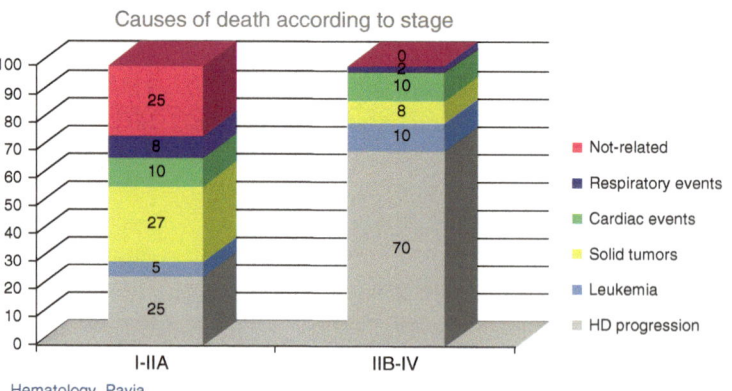

Fig. 3.4 Causes of death in early-stage (I–IIA) and advanced-stage (IIB–IVB) Hodgkin lymphoma according to Haematology Department of S. Matteo IRCCS Institute (Courtesy of E. Brusamolino)

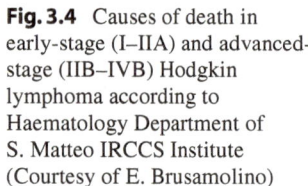

escalation in high-risk interim PET-positive, HL patients. In this review we will first review the phase II, already concluded studies and we will decribe then the outline and the preliminary results of the ongoing phase III trial based on a PET response-adapted strategy.

3.3.1   Phase II Concluded Studies in Early-Stage Disease

As soon as the prognostic role of interim PET scan to predict the final treatment outcome in early-stage HL became manifest [43], this strong therapy predictor was harnessed to answer the historical question revolving around the dilemma whether combined modality treatment with chemoradiation (CMT) should be preferred to chemotherapy alone for a deeper and immediate disease control in early-stage HL. The higher acute disease control, with a 3–7 % superior PFS, as shown in four published randomized clinical comparing CMT vs. chemotherapy alone in early-stage HL [61–64], did not translate to an improvement in OS of CMT. On the contrary, the final analysis of the National Cancer Institute of Canada Clinical Trials Group (NCIC-CTG) and Eastern Cooperative Oncology Group (ECOG) HD.6 study showed superior OS for chemotherapy alone at 12 years, due to increased late events/ toxicity in the CMT arm [65]. Similarly, the GHSG in the HD10/11 trials while showing an improved long-term disease control (8-y time to treatment failure) was unable to show an advantage in OS for patients treated with CMT as compared to chemotherapy alone [66]. On the other hand, clinicians should be cognizant of the fact that the scope of these trials was not merely to compare the treatment efficacy between the therapy arms but also to assess the benefits of omitting RT as a well-known risk factor for late toxicity. With the understanding that second-line treatments at the time of relapse can be quite effective in overcoming the transient survival disadvantage, RT can be probably safely avoided, at least in the patient subset with early favourable disease [17].

Due to very high NPV of interim PET in early-stage HL [8, 37, 38, 51, 67], its most attractive use in a PET response-adapted strategy in early-stage HL is likely the de-escalation of therapy either with chemotherapy abbreviation or even omitting radiotherapy. However compared to advanced-stage, data are less mature and results are controversial in early stage disease. The interest for the predictive value on interim PET scan was ignited in 2005 by Hutchings et al. in a pioneer retrospective study conducted in a cohort of 85 early and advanced HL patients undergoing interim PET after 2–3 cycles of ABVD; however, the positive predictive value of interim PET was much less evident in limited stage [43]. This lower predictive value could be largely explained by the concept that chemo-resistance does not imply a priori a refractoriness to radiation therapy, which is an essential part of the combined-modality treatment (CMT) in early-stage HL [28]. This concept has been elegantly proved by Sher et al. [67], who reported a 2-year failure-free survival of 92 % vs. 69 % for patients undergoing consolidation radiotherapy vs. no further treatment for patients with a mid-treatment positive PET scan after completion of the chemotherapy program.

In a prospective study aimed at assessing the effectiveness of the less toxic regimen with doxorubicin, vinblastine, and gemcitabine (AVG) compared to ABVD, early-stage HL patient underwent restaging with PET/CT after 2 and 6 cycles of chemotherapy [44]. After a mean follow-up of 3.3 years (0.4–5.0), the 2-year PFS for cycle 2 PET-negative and PET-positive patients were 88 % and 54 %, respectively, compared with 89 % and 27 % for cycle 6 PET-negative and PET-positive patients. The NPV and PPV for interim PET were 84.4 % and 45.8 %, respectively. This relatively low NPV could be explained by the lower effectiveness of AVG chemotherapy regimen compared to ABVD (CR rate 94 % vs. 81 %). The reasons for the disappointingly low PPV have been already reported, including the high patient rescue rate with radiation therapy.

Le Roux et al. reported the results of a PET-adapted strategy in a cohort of 90 HL patients in a perfect balance between early stage (45 patients) and advanced stage (45 patients), prospectively enrolled in a single institution [68]. After four cycles of ABVD, patients underwent a mid-treatment evaluation including CT and FDG PET/CT scan. Patients with negative FDG PET/CT or positive interim FDG PET/CT but in CR according to CT completed the pre-planned treatment for low-risk patients: IFRT for early favourable HL and additional or four more cycles of ABVD for early unfavourable and advanced stages (III and IV). Patients with positive interim FDG PET/CT but not in CR were addressed to autologous stem cell transplantation (ASCT). The criterion for a positive interim PET was a FDG uptake higher than background. In a following separate analysis, three different criteria for interim PET interpretation were than retrospectively used. After a median follow-up of 49 (13–81) months, 6 of 31 patients with a positive and 7 of 59 patients with a negative interim PET scan presented treatment failure. Again, the NPV was very high (95 %) and the PPV very low (16 %). Another prospective study was launched in Italy to assess the role of PET scan in guiding radiotherapy in both early- and advanced-stage patients in complete remission at the end of chemotherapy. One hundred-sixty HL patients with bulky disease at baseline defined as a node with a diameter >5 cm, showing a negative end-of-therapy PET scan after 6 courses of vinblastine, etoposide, bleomycin, epirubicin, and prednisone (VEBEP), were randomized to receive to radiotherapy or observation [69]. Two thirds of the patients in both arms had limited-stage disease (stage I-IIA). At 40-month median follow-up, PFS was 86 % in the chemotherapy arm compared to 96 % in the CMT arm, the difference being statistically significant ($p = .03$). The overall diagnostic accuracy of FDG PET to exclude impending relapses in the patients non-protected by radiotherapy was 86 % with a false-negative rate of 14 %. All the relapses in the chemotherapy only arm occurred in the bulky site and contiguous nodal regions. The largest concluded phase II study is the RAPID trial, on behalf of the UK National Cancer Research Institute (NCRI) [70]. The study enrolled 602 patients with non-bulky, early-stage (IA–IIA) disease with a median age of 34 years. Sixty-two percent of enrolled patients had a favourable prognosis according to EORTC criteria. Following three cycles of ABVD, an interim PET scan was performed (PET-3). 420 patients with a negative PET-3 were randomized to either no further therapy (NFT) or involved-field radiotherapy (IFRT): 209 to IFRT and 211 to NFT. Patients with a positive PET-3 were treated with a fourth ABVD cycle, followed by IFRT (Fig. 3.5).

Interim PET scan was interpreted according to the Deauville five-point scale [71], but the threshold for a positive scan was set between scores 2 and 3 ("sensitive" threshold), in order to avoid false-negative results. Seventy-five percent had a negative (scores 1–2) and 25 % a positive (scores 3–5) PET-3 scan. After a median follow-up of 60 months from randomization, in an intent-to-treat (ITT) analysis, PFS and OS were not statistically different between the arms. The 3-year progression-free survival rate was 94.6 % (95 % confidence interval [CI], 91.5–97.7) in the radiotherapy group and 90.8 % (95 % CI, 86.9–94.8) in the NFT group, with an absolute risk difference of −3.8 percentage points (95 % CI, −8.8 to 1.3). The trial was a non-inferiority, randomized study powered to exclude a ≥7 % difference in PFS of the experimental arm vs. the standard arm, and therefore the endpoint was met. However, in a per-protocol (PP) analysis, upon exclusion of 26 patients allocated to IFRT and not irradiated, 3-year PFS was 97.1 % for the IFRT arm and 90.8 % for the NFT arm. Moreover, as further confounding factor, all the 5 deaths recorded in the study occurred in patients allocated to IFRT arm, before starting radiation therapy.

Fig. 3.5 Final results of the UK NCRI RAPID trial: progression-free survival of irradiated vs. no further treatment patients. (**a**) progression-free survival for irradiated versus no further treatment patients: Intention to treat analysis. (**b**) progression-free survival for irradiated versus no further treatment patients: per-protocol analysis. (From Radford et al. [70])

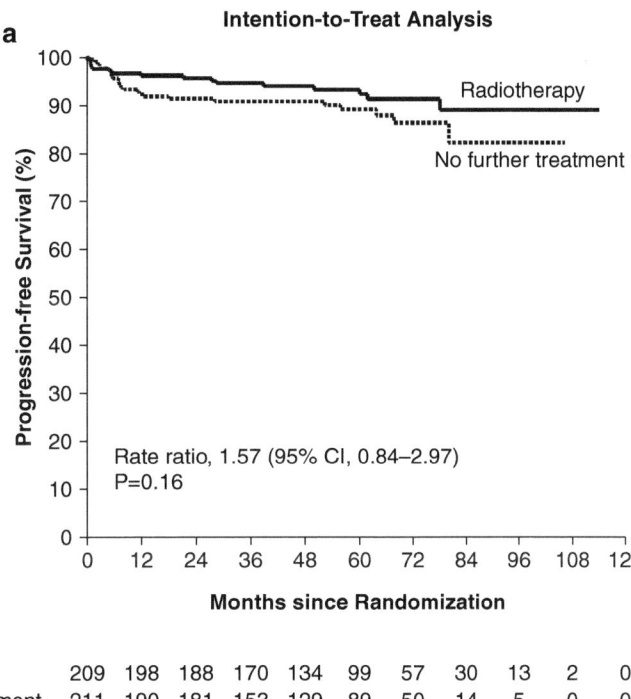

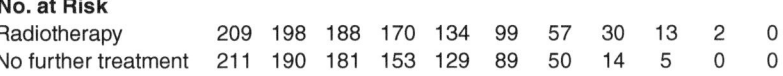

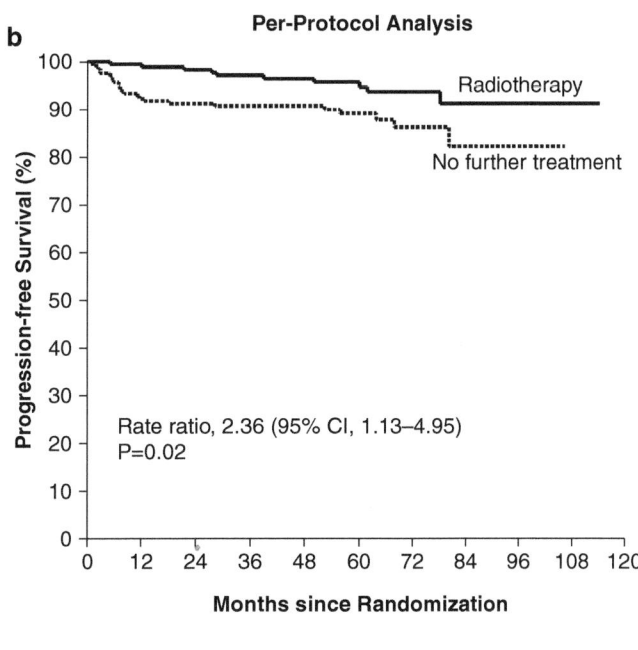

3.3.2 Phase II Ongoing Trials in Early-Stage Disease

Three European groups, EORTC (European Organization for Radiotherapy and Treatment of Cancer), LYSA (Lymphoma Study Association) and FIL (Italian Foundation on Lymphoma), jointly launched a prospective phase III PET response-adapted randomized study both in early favourable (H10F arm) and early unfavourable (H10U arm) HL. In this trial the interim PET was performed after 2 ABVD cycles (PET-2) and the scans were centrally reviewed. The endpoint was a non-inferiority of the experimental arm (PET-2-adapted strategy) compared to standard arm in both strata (3 ABVD+IFRT in H10F or 4 ABVD+IFRT in H10U, respectively, whatever the result of PET-2). Both in H10F and H10U, the experimental arm was split in an escalation arm and a de-escalation arm, according to PET-2 result: in the former, PET-2-positive patients are treated with 2 BEACOPP esc., followed by IFRT 20 Gy., irrespective of the risk stratum (both H10F and H10U). In the latter, PET-2-negative

patients are treated with 2 further ABVD (H10F) or 4 further ABVD (H10U) (see Fig. 3.6).

An interim futility analysis of the primary end point was scheduled after documentation of 12 and 22 events (progression, relapse, or death) for the H10 F and H10 U subgroups, respectively. The Deauville five-point scale was adopted as interpretation key for PET-2: the rate of PET-2 negative in the H10F and H10U studies was 86 % and 75 %, respectively. The recently published results of the pre-planned interim analysis led to opposite conclusions compared to RAPID study [72]. In the H10F stratum approximately 190 patients have been randomized to each study arm: 1 single event was recorded in the standard arm compared to 9 in the non-irradiated PET-2-negative arm. In the H10U study nearly 260 patients were randomized: 7 and 16 events occurred in the standard arm and in non-irradiated PET-2-negative arm, respectively. Based on the statistical analysis, despite the very low number of events, futility was declared ($p = .017$ and $.026$, respectively). The data safety and Monitoring Board amended the study by closing the experi-

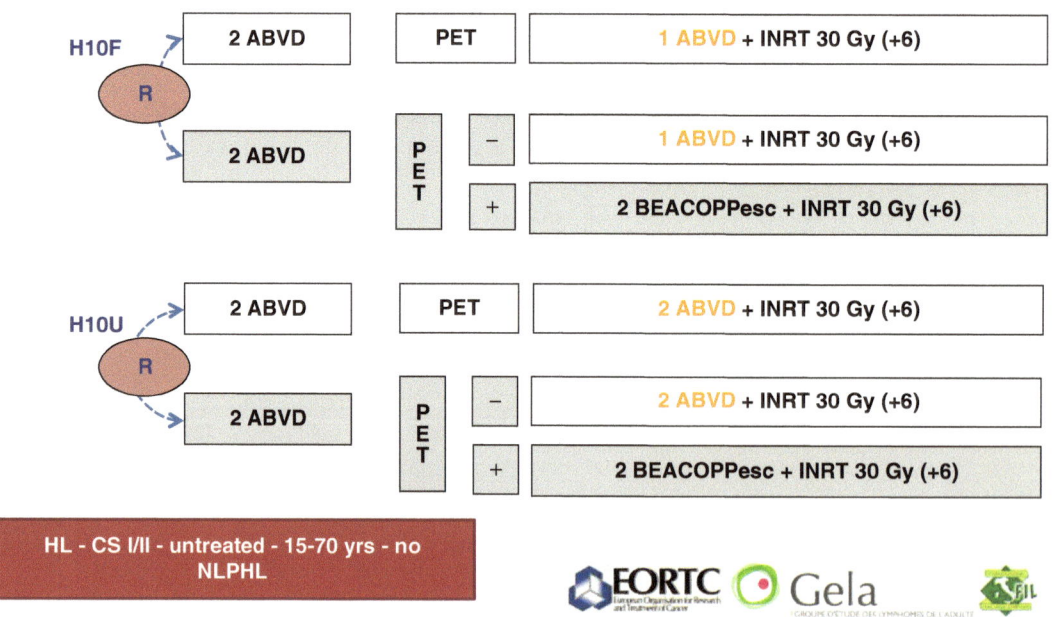

Fig. 3.6 The EORTC, LYSA, FIL H10 trial in early favourable and unfavourable Hodgkin lymphoma (From Raemaekers et al. [72])

mental, de-intensification arm. The results of the intensification arm have been recently presented during the 13th ICML in Lugano [73]. Briefly, 361/1950 (18 %) patients had a positive interim PET scan: 159 continued with one (H10F) or two (H10U) ABVD courses plus INRT, while 169 switched in both strata groups to BEACOPP escalated for two courses, followed by INRT. After a minimum follow-up of 4.5 years, the 5-y PFS was 77 % for ABVD vs. 91 % for the BEACOPP esc. arm ($p = .002$). However the 5-y OS showed only a non-significant superiority for the intensification arm: 89 % vs. 96 % ($p = .06$).

The German Hodgkin Study Group (GHSG) launched two prospective, non-inferiority clinical trials in favourable (HD 16) and unfavourable (HD 17) early-stage HL [74, 75]. The trials are similar in endpoint (non-inferiority study) and experimental design to the EORTC/LYSA/FIL H10 trial. In both trials a chemoradiation program non-PET-based with ABVD (HD 16) or BEACOPP (HD 17) and IFRT in the standard arm is compared to a chemotherapy-alone program in PET-2-negative patients and a CMT program with the corresponding chemotherapy regimen in PET-2-positive patients. Both studies were powered to a ≤5 % non-inferiority statistical design.

Two American collaborative groups, Cancer and Leukemia Group B and Eastern Cooperative Oncology Group, are conducting two very interesting trials in early-stage bulky HL, in which interim PET-positive patients after 2 ABVD courses are treated with 4 BEACOPP escalated cycles, followed by IFRT. The former trial is designed to omit INRT to the PET-2-negative subset [76] and the latter to deliver the conventional combination of ABVD + INRT to PET-negative patients [77].

3.3.3 Phase II Concluded Studies in Advanced-Stage Disease

In advanced-stage disease, a heated historical dilemma spanned over two decades to answer the following question: should a more effective treatment like escalated BEACOPP (EB) be indis-

criminately given to all patients at disease onset or could it be delivered only to those with relapsing or refractory disease after standard ABVD, with the intent of sparing undue toxicity to all the patient cohort [78]? Despite the proven superiority of EB over standard ABVD, in terms of 10-year PFS, which has been reported in four randomized clinical trials [56, 79–82], a large meta-analysis conducted on 2868 patients with advanced-stage HL concluded that there was no significant difference in OS between respective groups receiving either treatment [83]. Here again, as for limited disease, PET scan could ideally play the role of "arbiter" in this debate. As previously mentioned, early interim PET scan proved the most accurate predictor of treatment outcome in advanced-stage, ABVD-treated, HL patients [45].

Moving from these observations since 2006 onward, several Italian haematology institutions convened to adopt an interim PET response driven strategy in advance-stage HL patients, to prospectively validate the following working hypothesis: (1) if very high-risk PET-2-positive patients could be rescued with EB in at least half of cases and (2) if the overall outcome of the entire cohort of patients could be improved compared to standard historical results of ABVD treatment. The results of this study showed that after a median follow-up of 34 months (12–52), the 2-year failure-free survival (FFS) for the entire patient cohort was 91 %: 62 % for PET-2-positive and 95 % for PET-2-negative patients [84]. The working hypothesis was thus confirmed, and this therapeutic strategy proved feasible.

Similar to limited-stage HL, the therapy goal for advanced disease includes both maximizing treatment efficacy and avoiding undue toxicity for low-risk patients who do not require intensified therapies. Nevertheless, the primary treatment objective differs significantly from that of limited-stage HL, in that treatment intensification in high-risk disease takes precedence over minimizing therapy-related side effects. Both hypotheses, however, have been addressed in small phase II, single-centre or large cooperative multicentre clinical trials which have been recently concluded and published, adopting a escalation or a de-escalation strategy based on PET-2 result after ABVD or BEACOPP, respectively [85, 86]. While data from Ganesan [85] seem very similar to that reported in the interim analysis of other large multicentre trials with the same endpoint, Deau et al. reported the results of a retrospective analysis on a small cohort of 64 advanced-stage HL who were consecutively enrolled in a single institution in a time lag spanning over 6 years. Treatment started with 2 EB courses and patients had their treatment adapted in the basis of interim PET results [86]. Fifty-five patients (86%) achieved a negative PET-2. Six relapses (11%) occurred within the PET-2-negative group, mostly during the first year of follow-up (range: 4–14 months). In the PET-2-positive group, five patients showed disease progression with a positive PET after two more EB cycles (PET-4) and were allocated to salvage therapy. Moreover, four (44%) PET-2-positive patients relapsed. After a median follow-up of 30 months, the 2-year PFS was 87% in the PET-2-negative group but was only 47% in the PET-2-positive arm ($p = .0059$).

3.3.4 Phase II Ongoing Trials in Advanced-Stage Disease

Three large, international prospective multicentre trials sharing (a) the inclusion criteria, (b) the main study endpoint, (3) the interpretation key for interim PET (the Deauville five-point scale) and (4) the overall treatment strategy were launched in 2007 from US intergroup (S0816 trial), from UK National Cancer Research Institute (RATHL study) and from Italian Gruppo Italiano Terapie Innovative nei Linfomi (GITIL) and the Italian Foundation on Lymphoma (FIL), the HD0607 study [87–89]. The common trial backbone is the following: advanced-stage HL patients (IIB-IVB) are treated with two ABVD courses, and an interim PET is performed afterwards (PET-2). Patients showing a positive PET-2 switch to EB (minimum 4 courses) patients with a negative PET-2 continue with ABVD for a total of 6 cycles. Secondary intra-arm randomizations are planned

in the RATHL study (ABVD vs. AVD in PET-2-negative patients) and in the HD 0607 study (consolidation radiotherapy vs. no further treatment in PET-2-negative arm). Preliminary results from the interim analysis of these trials have been presented in abstract form. The preliminary results of the US intergroup trial S0816 on behalf of four cooperative groups have been presented at the twelfth ICML meeting of Lugano [90]. An overall population of 357 pts was available in whom interim PET-2 scan was centrally reviewed, and Deauville five-point scale was used to report the scans. Two-hundred-ninety-two patients (82%) were PET-negative (score 1–3) and 65 (18%) were PET-positive (scores 4–5). Out of 349 patients registered to continue therapy, based on the interim PET result, 291 continued with ABVD and 58 with EB. The Kaplan–Meier estimate for 1-year overall survival was 98% (95% CI: 95%, 99%) and for 1-year PFS was 84% (95% CI: 79%, 89%). The 1-year PFS of PET-2 negative and positive was 85% (95% CI: 79%, 90%) and 72%, respectively. The preliminary results of the RATHL study have been also presented during the 13th ICML in Lugano [91]. PET-2 results were available from 1137 patients with the following breakdown: 954 (84%) were negative and 183 (16%) positive. Among PET-2-negative pts, 65% of patients treated with ABVD and 69% of patients treated with AVD achieved CR or Cru. The CR/CRu rate was dependent on PET-2 Deauville five-point score: score 1, 82%; score 2, 72%; and score 3, 58% ($p < 0.01$). Those with positive PET-2 who received intensified therapy with EB reached a negative PET-3 in 74% of cases. The 3-year PFS for PET-2 patients treated with eBEACOPP or BEACOPP-14 and for PET-2 negative treated with ABVD or AVD was 66%, 82.5%, 85.4% and 84.4%, respectively. The 3-y PFS for the entire cohort of patient was 82.5% (80.1–84.7).

The results of the second interim analysis from the GITIL/FIL HD 0607 trial have also been presented in the same meeting [92]. The trial has been closed in June 2014: 753 patients have been enrolled and 656 (84%) completed the treatment. 114 (17.3%) had a positive, and 542 (82.6%) a negative PET-2 upon blinded independent central review (BICR). Treatment efficacy could be assessed in a cohort of 500 patients with a minimum follow-up of 2 years after the end of treatment of 1065.5 days (749.5–1299.5). A continuous complete remission (CCR) was recorded in 68 out of 97 PET-2-positive patients who switched to EB (70%) and in 351 out of 400 PET-2-negative patients (88%) who continued with ABVD. The probability of 2-y PFS and 5-y PFS were 66% and 62%, 89% and 85% and 84% and 81% for PET-2-positive, PET-2-negative and the overall cohort of patients, respectively ($p < .001$). In conclusion, more than 2000 patients have been enrolled in those three trials: therefore, critical information and new treatment options of these patients will be soon available. Importantly, the results of interim PET using the Deauville 5-point scale confirmed the reproducibility of this interpretation key across these studies: the percentages of PET-2-positive patients in this very large pool of patients from the UK, USA and Italian trials were 16%, 18% and 17%, respectively (see Table 3.3).

Although based on preliminary data, the following observations could be done: (1) nearly 10% of the PET-2-negative patients experience a treatment failure; this percentage seems twice that reported in previous non-adapted observational studies [8, 32, 37, 38, 43, 44, 46, 47]; (2) nearly two-thirds (60–70%) of the PET-2-positive patients could be rescued with EB and achieve a long-term remission. (3) The 2-year PFS of the overall cohort of patients seems slightly better than that obtained with standard ABVD treatment, with a gain in PFS of 5–10% compared to historical controls [53].

Another critical point is the procedure to adjudicate the final result or the PET scan review process. While no data are from the U.S. intergroup S0813 or from the RATHL studies, the Italian GITIL/FIL study adopted Blinded Independent Central Review procedure (BICR). Besides the decision that the local PET site must cede the final determination of a patient's status to the central review, which should bilaterally agreed between the sponsor and the local PET site, this choice depended on the need to check the reproducibility of the 5-point Deauville scale (5-PS)

and the agreement coefficient among reviewers [93]. The 5-PS for interim PET interpretation was just proposed at that time [71] and no validation studies were available on the reproducibility of those interpretation rules. Moreover, the U.S. Food and Drug Administration (FDA) recommends BICR for trials where reviewer's blinding is not achievable, and reviewers are informed that their decision would be determinant to decide a switch to a more aggressive treatment [94].

Finally, technological progress on the web-based imaging exchange and the availability of the web platform WIDEN® to upload and download images [95] have rendered BICR and the consequent treatment decision by the local clinical investigator possible and timely. In the HD0607 trial the median scan uploading and downloading times were 1 min, 25 s, and 1 min 55 s, respectively; the average and median times for central review were 47 h, 53 m, and 37 h, 43 m, respectively. The binary concordance between pairs of reviewers (Cohen's k) ranged from 0.72 to 0.85. The 5-point scale concordance among all reviewers was (Krippendorf alpha) was 0.77 [95].

At this writing no conclusive or preliminary data are available of clinical trials adopting a de-escalation strategy after EB, with the exception of the results of an interim analysis of the Israeli H2 trial [96], which has been presented during the 9th International Symposium on Hodgkin Lymphoma in Cologne [97]. Patients with advanced-stage HL are first assigned to therapy based on IPS score: IPS 0–2 receive 2 ABVD courses and IPS ≥ 3 two EB courses. An interim PET is performed afterwards in both strata: if PET-2 is negative, 4 more cycles of ABVD are given, followed by IFRT to bulky mediastinal masses. In PET-2-positive arm with no evidence of HL progression, 4 EB cycles are given, followed by IFRT on mediastinal bulky masses. Treatment de-escalation was possible in 80% of advanced-stage patients. No data are available on treatment escalation. At a median follow-up of 24 months (4–74), PFS was 82% for the entire cohort of advanced-stage patients. An overview of interim PET adapted clinical trials is provided in Fig. 3.7.

Trial Name	Sample	Stage	End-point	Before PET-2	PET-2 neg. arm	PET-2 pos. arm	PET Key Interpret.
Israeli H2	300	I-IV	3-y PFS	ABVDx2	ABVDx4	EBx4 HD+ASCT	Dynamic score
AHL (LYSA)	798	IIB-IVB	5-y PFS	EBx2	EB x 6 ABVDx2	EBx6	5-PS
HD 18 (GHSG)	1500	IIB-IVB	5-Y PFS	EBx2	EB x 6 ABVDx4	EBx6 ±R	5-PS^m
HD 0607 (FIL/GITIL)	750	IIB-IVB	3-y PFS	ABVDx2	ABVDx4 +/- RT	EBx2 + BB x 4	5-PS
RATHL (NCRI)	1200	II-IVB	3-y PFS	ABVDx2	ABVDx4 AVD x 4	EBx4 B-14 x 6	5-PS
S0813 (SWOG-CALGB)	230	III-IVB	2-y PFS	ABVDx2	ABVDx4	EBx6 Bx6 (HIV+)	5-PS
HD 0801 (FIL)	300	IIB-IVB	2-y PFS	ABVDx2	ABVDx4 +/- RT	IGEVx4+ ASCT	IHP

Fig. 3.7 Overview of the PET-adapted clinical trials in advanced-stage HL. *EB* escalated BEACOPP, *R* rituximab, *RT* consolidation radiotherapy, *LYSA* Lymphoma Study group de l'Adulte, *GHSG* German Hodgkin Lymphoma Study Group, *FIL* Italian Foundation on Lymphoma, *GITIL* Italian: Group For Innovative Therapy of Lymphoma, *NCRI* National Cancer Research Institute, *SWOG* South Western Oncology Group, *CALGB* Cancer and Acute Leukemia Group

3.4 PET to Guide Consolidation Radiotherapy

One of the most compelling applications of PET imaging in HL has been guiding consolidation radiotherapy for residual mass persisting after chemotherapy.

Tumour bulk decreases over time during cytostatic treatment, and the rationale for using FDG PET for chemotherapy response assessment is based on the strong relationship between FDG uptake entity and cancer cell number, which has been reported in a substantial number of studies [98, 99]. Therefore, a decline in FDG uptake during tumour shrinkage results from reduction of the number of viable neoplastic cells, while a sustained increase of SUV values is seen upon tumour regrowth. On the other hand, the relationship between a CT-detected tumour mass and clinical response could be lost in chemo-sensitive neoplastic disorders, as the metabolic slowdown of the neoplastic tissue could precede by months the reduction of

tumour volume. As a consequence, 60–80 % of HL patients show a residual mass during end-of-treatment restaging mostly in sites of bulky disease recorded at baseline [5, 6], but only less than half of these masses still harbour residual disease [100]. This phenomenon was first described in lymphoma entering a sustained clinical remission at the end of therapy, but later it has also been reported in a number of solid tumours such as head and neck squamous cell carcinoma (HNSCC) and gastrointestinal stromal tumours (GIST), in whom a metabolic response of the tumour, documented by a negative FDG PET/CT scan, invariably preceded the anatomical response detected on CT [101, 102].

In pre-PET era, Bonadonna et al. in Milan originally proposed a boost of consolidation RT for bulky nodal lesions or residual masses in advanced HL as an integral part of ABVD treatment [53]. However, with the advent of PET, it became possible to discriminate residual active disease from fibrotic tissue at the end of chemotherapy in lymphoma, with a sensitivity of

43–100 % and a specificity of 67–100 % [103]. Owing to its ability to detect persisting viable tissue, functional imaging with PET/CT proved superior to conventional radiological in defining the prognosis of tumour masses detected at the end of chemotherapy and turned out an ideal tool for guiding consolidation radiotherapy. Predictably, the NPV of the end-treatment PET depends on the efficacy of the administered chemotherapy, being as high as 94 % with very effective chemotherapy regimens such as EB [104] or as low as 75 % after the low-intensity VEBEP regimen [69, 105].

A very elegant and convincing demonstration of these concepts came from the results of the large HD15 trial of the GHSG, in whom consolidation radiotherapy was administered only to advanced-stage HL patients, showing a PET-positive, CT-detected residual mass with a diameter ≥ 2.5 cm at the end of three different EB regimens. The 4-year PFS of irradiated vs. non-irradiated patients was 86.2 % and 92.6 %, respectively ($P = 0.022$). The NPV of end-therapy PET was as high as 94 %. A residual mass was detected by CT scan in 739/2126 (34.7 %) and 191 out of these 739 (26 %) had a positive PET scan at the end of treatment [104]. A very important conclusion of the trial was that consolidation radiotherapy was needed only for 11 % of the enrolled patients compared to 71 % in the HD 9 trial [56]. In a subsequent analysis, combining dimensional data of the residual mass (i.e. measuring the largest diameter of the residual lesion in trans-axial CeCT slices) with PET/CT data, the same group was able to refine and improve the interpretation criteria of end-of-therapy scan to predict treatment outcome, by measuring the dimension of the residual mass: in the PET-positive patients a decrease in size of the residual mass $\geq 65\%$ from baseline values decreased the false-negative results [106].

Similar conclusions have been reached in a cohort of ABVD-treated advanced-stage patients by Savage et al. on behalf of the British Columbia Cancer Agency (BCCA) and reported in abstract form [107]. All the advanced-stage HL patients enrolled in clinical trials on behalf of BCCA after 2005 showing a residual mass at CT scan

with a diameter ≥ 2 cm. at the end of ABVD treatment and a negative PET scan, the consolidation radiotherapy was omitted. In short, 151 patients with advanced stage HL and a PET-negative residual mass at the end of treatment had a 5-year progression-free survival of 92 %, and a subset of 71 patients with a PET-negative residual mass in a nodal region where a bulky lesion with a diameter ≥ 10 cm was recorded at baseline had a 5-y PFS of 90 %. The overall NPV and PPV of end-of-therapy PET scan were 92 % and 55 %, respectively. This study confirmed the high NPV of end-of therapy PET scan in patients treated with adequate-intensity chemotherapy regimen. The low positive predictive value could be due to the rescue treatment with consolidation radiotherapy but also to false-positive PET scan results due to an unspecific tissue inflammation secondary to chemotherapy-induced tumour lysis [108]. In conclusion, the decision to irradiate a single PET-positive residual mass should be taken in the awareness of false-positive results especially in the case of residual masses showing a dramatic shrink compared to baseline dimensions.

3.5 PET During Second-Line Treatment

The standard therapeutic option for second-line treatment of relapsed or refractory HL is high-dose chemotherapy (HDT), followed by autologous haematopoietic stem cell transplantation (ASCT), resulting in a rescue and long-term disease control in up of two-thirds of patients. Successful outcome depends on remission duration after first-line chemotherapy and chemosensitivity to second-line or salvage therapy prior to ASCT [109, 110]. Furthermore, recent meta-analysis data confirmed the prognostic value of pre-ASCT FDG PET imaging in lymphoma, demonstrating a poor long-term disease control in PET-positive patients after induction chemotherapy (31–41 %) compared with a PFS of 73–82 % in those who achieved a PET-negative remission before undergoing HDT/ASCT [111–114]. Moving from these observations, a PET response-adapted strategy was also proposed during second-line rescue treatment including HDT and ASCT for relapsing/refractory HL. In a non-randomised, open-label, single-centre, phase 2 trial, 45 patients refractory to doxorubicin-containing first-line treatment received weekly infusions of 1.2 mg/kg brentuximab vedotin (BV) on days 1, 8, and 15 for two 28-day cycles. After completion of two cycles, patients received a PET scan. Twelve patients (27%, 95% CI 13–40) were PET-negative, with a Deauville score 1 or 2, and proceeded straight to HDT/ASCT, while 33 (73%, 95% CI 60–86) were PET-positive (Deauville 3–5) after BV. One still PET-positive patient withdrew consent, and therefore 32 PET-positive patients received HDT with augmented ICE (ifosfamide 5000 mg/m^2 in combination with mesna 5000 mg/m^2, continuous infusion every 12 h, days 1 and 2; carboplatin, single dose AUC 5, day 3; etoposide 200 mg/m^2 every 8 h, day 1 for three doses), for two cycles. After HDT PET scan reverted to negativity in 22/32 (69%, 95% C.I. 53–85) cases. Overall, 34/45 patients (76%, 95% CI 62–89) achieved PET negativity [115]. However due to the very short number of enrolled patient and the very short follow-up (nearly 1 year after treatment end), these observations should be taken with caution and considered preliminary, to be confirmed in a larger phase III trial. Interestingly, a very conservative cut-off value for a negative scan (score ≤ 2) was adopted along the 5-PS. This choice, as in other clinical trials as the RAPID study [70] aimed at assessing the role of interim PET for treatment de-escalation, was adopted in order to maximize the sensitivity of the imaging technique, as recently proposed in the Lugano Workshop on PET scan for lymphoma staging and restaging [116]. Different from the abundant historical data present in the literature in front-line treatment prediction, very few reports are available on the predictive value of interim PET scan during salvage therapy. In a small cohort of 24 relapsing or refractory HL patients treated with rescue chemotherapy consisting of ifosfamide, gemcitabine and vinorelbine (IGEV) followed by ASCT, PET scan was predictive of final treatment outcome when performed after the sec-

ond cycle. The 2-year PFS was 93% vs. 10% for patients with PET-negative and PET-positive results, respectively ($P < 0.001$) [117]. More recently, brentuximab vedotin (BV) turned out as the most active drug for relapsing refractory HL, proving able to induce an overall response rate (ORR) as high as 75% in HL patients treated with up to 13 lines of chemotherapy [118, 119]. BV is an antibody-drug conjugate composed of the anti-CD30 chimeric immunoglobulin G1 (IgG1) monoclonal antibody cAC10 conjugated with the potent anti-microtubule drug monomethyl auristatin E (MMAE) connected by a protease-cleavable linker; the drug is internalized in the HRS cells, which are selectively killed by the MMAE toxin. Several retrospective experiences have been reported with the use of BV in the so-called national-named patient program (NNP) for the compassionate use of BV in refractory HL, and interim PET was usually performed after 2–4 doses of BV administration. In the GHSG experience, 12 consecutive, heavily pretreated patients with relapsed and refractory HL treated with BV at the dose 1.8 mg/kg every 21 days were available for analysis. Interim PET was performed after a median of 3 cycles (range, 2–5 cycles) and was analysed visually using a 5-point scale (5PS). The 1-year PFS was 100% and 38% in patients with negative and positive interim PET, respectively ($p = 0.033$) [120]. Similar results were obtained in the Italian NNP in a retrospective study including 65 patients treated with a median number of 4 (2–13) prior cancer-related systemic regimens including HDT and ASCT or allogeneic stem cell transplant, receiving BV at the dose of 1.8 mg/kg every 21 days. In the absence of specific indications, response was assessed by PET/CT scans after cycles 3 and 8 (PET-3, PET-8) and at treatment discontinuation, according to the International Harmonization Program (IHP) criteria [121]. The best overall response rate (70.7%), including 21.5% complete responses, was observed at the first restaging after the third cycle of treatment (PET-3). Before the second interim evaluation, which was scheduled after eight cycles of BV (PET-8), 21 patients discontinued BV treatment: 12 of them for progressive disease and 3 for toxicity, while 6 underwent stem cell transplantation. The final response of the whole sample was as follows: 14 complete responses (21.5%), 5 partial responses (7.7%), 6 cases of stable disease and 40 cases of progressive disease. After a median follow-up of 13.2 months, the overall survival rate at 20 months was 73.8%, while the progression-free survival was 24.2% [122].

3.6 PET Scan Interpretation

3.6.1 Historical Proposal

In the pre-PET era, at the end of millennium, a first proposal for treatment response assessment in HL and non-Hodgkin lymphoma (NHL), based on traditional, radiological imaging, was proposed, with the aim of harmonizing the CT interpretation rules, later called the IWC (International workshop criteria) rules [123]. The latter were mainly based on the reduction of the nodal and extra-nodal lesion size. Cheson et al. included anatomic definitions of complete response, defined by a "normal" lymph node size defined as equal or lower than 1.5 cm in the longest transverse diameter in trans-axial slices of CT. A designation of complete response/unconfirmed (RCu) was adopted to include patients with radiological evidence of a residual mass at the end of treatment, showing a reduction on the largest diameter $\geq 75\%$ of that measured at baseline in the same mass. Partial response (PR) was defined a reduction in sum of the largest diameter of all the measurable nodal masses and extra-nodal lesions $\geq 50\%$ and stable disease (SD) of all the measurable nodal masses and extra-nodal lesions $\leq 25\%$. Progressive disease (PD) was defined as an increase in sum of the largest diameter of all the measurable nodal masses and extra-nodal lesions $> 50\%$ or new lesion.

In 2007, the exponential increase of PET use in lymphoma staging and restaging led to a revision of the IWC criteria by including PET/CT in the recommended panoply of imaging tools for treatment response assessment. On the other hand, specific rules for PET scan were also required, as it became clear that a residual FDG uptake at the end of treatment does not necessary mean persisting active disease [43]. New established criteria, the so-called International Harmonization Project criteria (IHP criteria), were therefore proposed for treatment response assessment in HL and NHL, based on literature data and consensus expert opinion [121]. The main points of the recommendations were the following:

- Baseline FDG PET (before treatment) was not deemed mandatory for FDG-avid lymphoma subtype Hodgkin Lymphoma (HL), diffuse large B-cell lymphoma (DLBCL), follicular lymphoma (FL), mantle cell lymphoma (MCL), but nevertheless recommended, to ease the end-of-treatment scan interpretation. In case of variably FDG-avid lymphoma, baseline PET was also recommended (e.g. peripheral T-cell lymphoma, marginal zone lymphoma).
- Patients had to be scanned at least 3 weeks, but preferably 6–8 weeks, after chemotherapy or chemo-immunotherapy end, and 8–12 weeks after radiation.
- Visual assessment alone was considered adequate for PET interpretation.
- Mediastinal blood pool activity was recommended as the reference background activity to compare the residual FDG uptake in case of a residual mass ≥ 2 cm in largest transverse diameter, regardless of its location.
- In case of a lesion with a lower-size residual mass (with the largest $\xi \leq 2$ cm), the lesion could be considered positive if its residual FDG uptake showed an intensity above that of the surrounding background.

Specific criteria for defining PET positivity in the liver, spleen, lung, and bone marrow were also proposed. The above criteria were then integrated in the revised response criteria of IWC [124], which included PET/CT and bone marrow biopsy data (Table 3.2).

More recently new criteria for interim and end-of-treatment PET scan interpretation have been proposed by experts, moving from the

Table 3.2 IHP criteria

Response	Definition	Nodal masses	Spleen, liver	Bone marrow
Complete remission (CR)	Disappearance of all evidence of disease	(a) FDG-avid or PET-positive prior to therapy; mass of any size permitted if PET-negative (b) Variably FDG-avid or PET-negative; regression to normal size on CT	Not palpable, nodules disappeared	Infiltrate cleared on repeat biopsy; if indeterminate by morphology, immunohistochemistry should be negative
Partial remission (PR)	Regression of measurable disease and no new sites	$\geq$50 % decrease in SPD of up to 6 largest dominant masses; no increase in size of other nodes (a) FDG-avid or PET-positive prior to therapy; one or more PET-positive at previously involved site (b) Variably FDG-avid or PET-negative; regression on CT	$\geq$50 % decrease in SPD of nodules (for single nodule in greatest transverse diameter); no increase in size of liver or spleen	Irrelevant if positive prior to therapy; cell type should be specified
Stable disease (SD)	Failure to attain CR/PR or PD	(a) FDG-avid or PET-positive prior to therapy; PET-positive at prior sites of disease and no new sites on CT or PET (b) Variably FDG-avid or PET-negative; no change in size of previous lesions on CT		
Relapsed disease or progressive disease (PD)	Any new lesion or increase by $\geq$50 % of previously involved sites from nadir	Appearance of a new lesion(s) >1.5 cm in any axis, $\geq$50 % increase in SPD of more than one node, or $\geq$50 % increase in longest diameter of a previously identified node >1 cm in short axis Lesions PET-positive if FDG-avid lymphoma or PET-positive prior to therapy	>50 % increase from nadir in the SPD of any previous lesions	New or recurrent involvement

SPD sum of the product of the diameters

following observations: (1) the low reproducibility of dimensional criteria in a lesion measured in trans-axial slices of CT scan, (2) the inconsistencies of FDG activity measure in small lesion due to the partial volume effect, and (3) the revised concept of minimal residual uptake (MRU), which was considerably widened to encompass a persisting FDG uptake with an intensity as high as that measured in the liver, far beyond that originally proposed by Hutchings et al. [43].

During the 1st international workshop on PET scan in lymphoma, held in Deauville (France) and the ensuing meetings in Menton (France), a visual five-point scale (so-called Deauville criteria, *detailed in the next paragraph*) was proposed and validation studies for these rules launched [125, 126].

The main challenge of the interim PET interpretation is based on the presence of a residual FDG uptake in interim and end-of-treatment PET scan which was deemed by nuclear medicine physicians non-disease-related: the so-called "minimal residual uptake" (MRU). The latter, according to the original Hutchings definition, was defined as low-grade uptake of FDG (just above background) in a focus within an area of previously noted disease reported by the nuclear medicine physicians as not likely to represent malignancy" [43]. This was recorded in the 10.6% of patients scanned after 2 or 3 courses of chemotherapy. However, the tumour shrinkage during chemotherapy is a continuous process, and PET scan is no longer able to detect tumour lesion with a diameter lower than 4–5 mm, which correspond to a reduction in tumour cell number of only two logarithms, but is still compatible with the presence of residual viable cells. It is therefore conceivable, at least in theory, that a residual FGD uptake could be a harbinger of residual viable neoplastic tissue. Moving from this assumption, new criteria incorporating PET (PERCIST) have been proposed moving from the traditional radiological response criteria in solud tumours (RECIST) have been proposed [127]. A residual uptake may therefore correspond to a residual disease, which would be just above this detectability threshold (Fig. 3.8).

However, due to the high chemosensitivity of lymphoma, the persistence of a single spot of residual FDG uptake in these neoplasms is nearly always due to a post-therapeutic inflammatory change. The MRU concept then evolved over time, with the aim of increase the specificity and the PPV of interim and final PET scan, as synthetized by Gallamini et al. [128] (Fig. 3.9).

As earlier mentioned, in 2005, Hutchings et al. defined a minimal residual uptake as a low FDG uptake, slightly higher than surrounding background, in a localization initially involved by lymphoma; this residual uptake was considered as probably non-malignant [43]. The significance of this observation stayed undetermined; the hypothesis was that it was due to unspecific FDG uptake by inflammatory cells infiltrating the tumour in response to chemotherapy. In this pioneer study, only one patient relapsed among the 9 patients with MRU at interim PET. In 2007, Juweid et al. defined MRU as a residual FDG uptake with intensity equal to mediastinal blood pool for lesion having a diameter equal or superior than 2 cm and with an intensity equal to background for lesions with a lower size (MBP) [121]. At the same time, Gallamini et al. defined MRU as low and persistent FDG uptake with intensity equal or slightly higher to MBP [8]. In 2008, Barrington et al. [129] defined MRU as residual uptake with intensity equal or lower than liver uptake. The concept of MRU has evolved

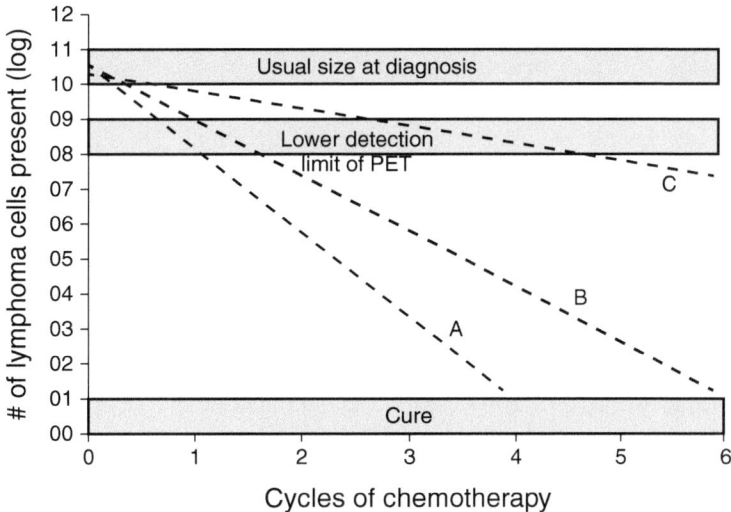

Fig. 3.8 The relation between different kinetics of tumour cell kill and the detection power of PET. (Extract from: From RECIST to PERCIST: Evolving Considerations for PET response criteria in solid tumours [127])

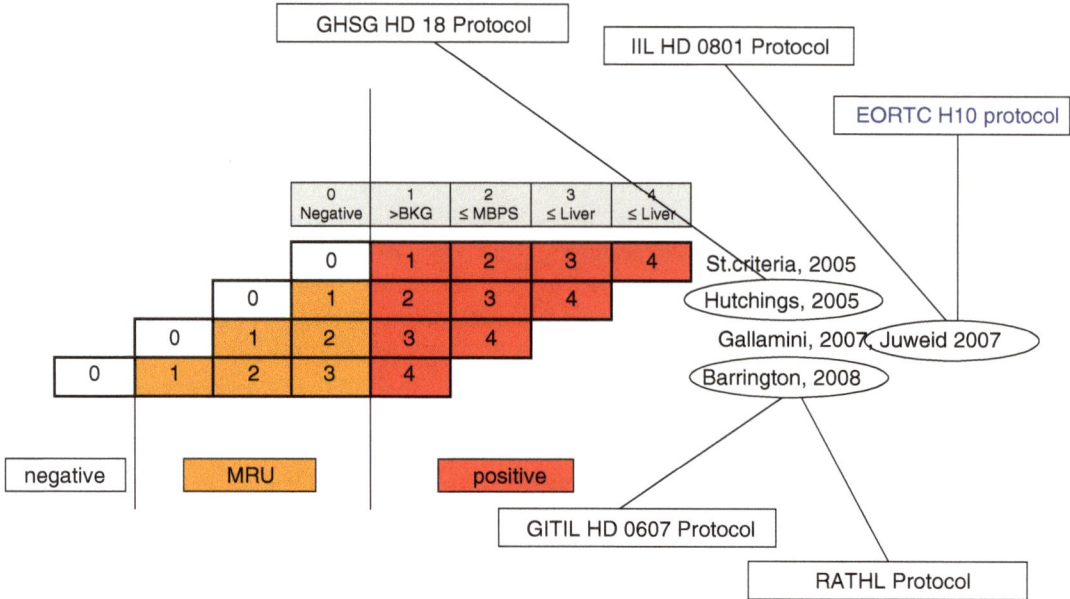

Fig. 3.9 The evolution of the MRU definition over time (From: Gallamini et al. [128]). *BKG* surrounding background, *MBPS* mediastinal blood pool structures, *MRU* minimal residual uptake

over time to include all the situations in which FDG uptake could be predictably attributed to an unspecific tissue reaction. Accordingly, the proposed threshold for a positive scan has been substantially raised. Moreover, different thresholds according to different clinical situations may be set. For example, for good prognosis patients, if the aim of a trial is a safe treatment de-escalation, a "sensitive" threshold with a high NPV is desirable. On the other hand, if the aim is intensifying treatment in interim-positive patients, a high PPV is requested for the interim scan, in order to spare patients with a predictably favourable outcome the undue toxicity of an aggressive therapy. [129]. Furthermore, Barrington et al. were able to demonstrate a fairly high inter-observer concordance when a threshold higher than liver uptake was used. All the above recommendations have been proposed during the first international workshop on interim PET in lymphoma held in Deauville (France) in April 2009, which was attended by haematologists and nuclear medicine experts in lymphoma [71]. The purpose of this meeting was to reach a consensus on simple and reproducible interpretation rules for interim PET

in HL and DLBCL and to launch two or more international validation studies (IVS) to validate these criteria.

The main conclusions of this workshop were the following:

- The threshold should be determined regarding clinical and therapeutic strategy, lymphoma subtypes and escalation or de-escalation therapeutic changes.
- The residual FDG uptake should be scored as follows:

1. No uptake
2. Uptake ≤ the mediastinum
3. Uptake > the mediastinum but ≤ the liver
4. Moderately increase uptake > the liver
5. Markedly increased uptake > the liver and/or new lesions related to lymphoma

- A visual analysis using a five-point scale (5-PS) is recommended, with MBP and the liver as reference points.

In April 2010, during the second international workshop PET in lymphoma "which was held in Menton (France), [130] the preliminary results of the application of the 5-point Deauville scale (5-PS) were presented and the problems in practical application discussed. In September 2011, during the Third International Workshop on PET in Lymphoma" [125], the final results of the international validation study (IVS) in Hodgkin lymphoma and diffuse large B-cell (DLBCL) lymphoma have been presented [131]. The results confirmed the prognostic value of interim PET in HL (PFS: 28 % in positive interim PET group vs. 95 % in negative interim PET group; $p < 0.0001$) and the reliability and reproducibility of Deauville five-point scale. The threshold chosen for a positive scan was between scores 3 and 4, with scores 1–3 considered as negative. The inter-observer agreement was very high (97 %). Forty-five patients out of 260 patients (17 %) showed a positive interim scan; however in 12 of them a false-positive result was recorded, upon central review of the scans. Nonetheless, a preliminary consensus was reached on the use of 5-PS for interim PET in HL, with a cutoff value for a positive scan between score 3 and 4. Finally, during the two last workshops in Menton (4th and 5th international workshop on PET in lymphoma, October 2012 and September 2014), the 5-PS was proposed also for other NHL subsets for interim and end-of-treatment PET scan interpretation [126, 132]. Some issues were still discussed, like: (a) the interest, the significance and the reproducibility of differentiating Deauville scores 4 and 5, (b) the different patterns of FDG uptake in bone marrow across NHL subtype and its respective clinical significance in relationship with the "gold standard" to assess bone marrow involvement by lymphoma (trephine bone marrow biopsy), (c) the visual reference organ to be used in case of liver disease, and (d) the significance of complete metabolic response with residual mass on CT. Preliminary reports of the use of quantitative PET scan (Q-PET) using standardized uptake value (SUV) and SUV-derived quantitative metrics, such as metabolic tumour volume (MTV) or total lesion glycolysis (TLG) have been also presented, but these results were considered as true preliminary and difficult to interpret owing to the complete absence of a program for Q-PET result standardization.

3.7 Current PET Interpretation Recommendations in Treatment Response Evaluation

The last updated recommendations including interim and end-of-treatment PET interpretation, and, more in general, for PET integration in the diagnostic workup for lymphoma staging and restaging, were agreed among nuclear medicine experts and clinicians convening in a closed workshop on PET scan in lymphoma during the 12th International Congress on Malignant Lymphoma (ICML) held in 2013 in Lugano. They are better known as "Lugano criteria for interim and end-of-treatment PET scan interpretation in Lymphoma" [133] (Table 3.3). The recommendations from this session could be displayed as follows:

3.7.1 Staging Procedures

- "Excisional biopsy is preferred for diagnosis, although core-needle biopsy may suffice when biopsy is not feasible.
- Clinical evaluation includes careful history, relevant laboratory tests, and recording of disease-related symptoms.
- PET-CT is the standard for FDG-avid lymphomas, whereas CT is indicated for non-avid lymphoma subsets.
- A modified Ann Arbor staging system is recommended", simply based on only two subsets with different tumour burden: early stage (Ann Arbor stages I or II, non-bulky) or advanced disease (Ann Arbor stages III or IV), with stage II bulky disease considered limited or advanced as determined by histology and a number of prognostic factors. This two-classes classification was not intended as guidance to treatment: patients should be treated according to prognostic and risk factors in each lymphoma subset.
- Suffixes A and B are only required for HL.
- The designation X for bulky disease is no longer necessary; instead, a recording of the largest tumor diameter is required.
- If a PET-CT is performed, a BMB is no longer indicated for HL; a BMB is only needed for DLBCL if the PET is negative and identifying a discordant histology is important for patient management".

Table 3.3 Lugano criteria for interim and end-of-treatment PET scan interpretation in Lymphoma [133]

Response and site	PET/CT-based response	CT-based response
Complete:	**Complete metabolic response:**	**Complete radiologic response** (all of the following):
Lymph nodes and extra-lymphatic sites	*Score 1, 2, or 3*[a] with or without a residual mass on 5PS	Target nodes/nodal masses must regress to ≤1.5 cm in LDi
	It is recognized that in Waldeyer's ring or extranodal sites with high physiologic uptake or with activation within spleen or marrow (e.g. with chemotherapy or myeloid colony-stimulating factors), uptake may be greater than normal mediastinum and/or liver. In this circumstance, complete metabolic response may be inferred if uptake at sites of initial involvement is no greater than the surrounding normal tissue even if the tissue has high physiologic uptake	No extra-lymphatic sites of disease
Non-measured lesion	Not applicable	Absent
Organ enlargement	Not applicable	Regress to normal
New lesions	None	None
Bone marrow	No evidence of FDG-avid disease in marrow	Normal by morphology; if indeterminate, IHC negative
Partial:	**Partial metabolic response:**	**Partial remission** (all of the following):
Lymph nodes and extra-lymphatic sites	*Score 4 or 5 with reduced uptake compared with baseline* and residual mass(es) of any size	≥50 % decrease in SPD of up to 6 target measurable nodes and extranodal sites
	At interim, these findings suggest responding disease	When a lesion is too small to measure on CT, assign 5 mm × 5 mm as the default value
	At end of treatment, these findings indicate residual disease	When no longer visible, 0 × 0 mm
		For a node >5 mm × 5 mm, but smaller than normal, use actual measurement for calculation
Non-measured lesion	Not applicable	Absent/normal, regressed, but no increase
Organ enlargement	Not applicable	Spleen must have regressed by >50 % in length beyond normal
New lesions	None	None
Bone marrow	Residual uptake higher than uptake in normal marrow but reduced compared with baseline (diffuse uptake compatible with reactive changes from chemotherapy allowed). If there are persistent focal changes in the marrow in the context of a nodal response, consideration should be given to further evaluation with MRI or biopsy or an interval scan	Not applicable
No response or stable disease:	**No metabolic response:**	**Stable disease:**
Target nodes/nodal masses, extranodal lesions	*Score 4 or 5 with no significant change in FDG uptake* from baseline at interim or end of treatment	<50 % decrease from baseline in SPD of up to 6 dominant, measurable nodes and extranodal sites; no criteria for progressive disease are met
Non-measured lesion	Not applicable	No increase consistent with progression
Organ enlargement	Not applicable	No increase consistent with progression

Table 3.3 (continued)

Response and site	PET/CT-based response	CT-based response
New lesions	None	None
Bone marrow	No change from baseline	Not applicable
Progressive disease:	**Progressive metabolic disease:**	**Progressive disease** requires at least 1 of the following PPD progression:
Individual target nodes/ nodal masses	*Score 4 or 5 with an increase in intensity of uptake* from baseline and/or	An individual node/lesion must be abnormal with:
Extranodal lesions	*New FDG-avid foci* consistent with lymphoma at interim or end-of-treatment assessment	LDi > 1.5 cm and Increase by ≥50 % from PPD nadir and An increase in LDi or SDi from nadir: 0.5 cm for lesions ≤2 cm 1.0 cm for lesions >2 cm In the setting of splenomegaly, the splenic length must increase by >50 % of the extent of its prior increase beyond baseline (e.g. a 15-cm spleen must increase to >16 cm). If no prior splenomegaly, must increase by at least 2 cm from baseline New or recurrent splenomegaly
Non-measured lesion	Not applicable	New or clear progression of pre-existing non measured lesions
New lesions	New FDG-avid foci consistent with lymphoma rather than another aetiology (e.g. infection, inflammation). If uncertain regarding aetiology of new lesions, biopsy or interval scan may be considered	Regrowth of previously resolved lesions A new node >1.5 cm in any axis A new extranodal site >1.0 cm in any axis; if <1.0 cm in any axis, its presence must be unequivocal and must be attributable to lymphoma Assessable disease of any size unequivocally attributable to lymphoma
Bone marrow	New or recurrent FDG-avid foci	New or recurrent involvement

Abbreviations: *5PS* 5-point scale, *CT* computed tomography, *FDG* fluoro-deoxy-glucose, *IHC* immunohistochemistry, *LDi* longest transverse diameter of a lesion, *MRI* magnetic resonance imaging, *PET* positron emission tomography, *PPD* cross product of the LDi and perpendicular diameter, *SDi* shortest axis perpendicular to the LDi, *SPD* sum of the product of the perpendicular diameters for multiple lesions

[a]A score of 3 in many patients indicates a good prognosis with standard treatment, especially if at the time of an interim scan. However, in trials involving PET where de-escalation is investigated, it may be preferable to consider a score of 3 as inadequate response (to avoid undertreatment). Measured dominant lesions: Up to six of the largest dominant nodes, nodal masses, and extranodal lesions selected to be clearly measurable in two diameters. Nodes should preferably be from disparate regions of the body and should include, where applicable, mediastinal and retroperitoneal areas. Non-nodal lesions include those in solid organs (e.g. the liver, spleen, kidneys, lungs), those with GI involvement, cutaneous lesions, or those noted on palpation. Non-measured lesions: Any disease not selected as measured, dominant disease and truly assessable disease should be considered not measured. These sites include any nodes, nodal masses, and extranodal sites not selected as dominant or measurable or that do not meet the requirements for measurability but are still considered abnormal, as well as truly assessable disease, which is any site of suspected disease that would be difficult to follow quantitatively with measurement, including pleural effusions, ascites, bone lesions, leptomeningeal disease, abdominal masses, and other lesions that cannot be confirmed and followed by imaging. In Waldeyer's ring or in extranodal sites (e.g. GI tract, liver, bone marrow), FDG uptake may be greater than in the mediastinum with complete metabolic response, but should be no higher than surrounding normal physiologic uptake (e.g. with marrow activation as a result of chemotherapy or myeloid growth factors)

3.7.2 Restaging Procedures

The 5-point scale (Deauville score) should be used for interim and end-of-treatment PET scan interpretation, both in clinical trials and in the daily clinical practice [116].

- PET/CT is used to assess early treatment response and, at end of treatment, to establish remission status.
- A score of 1 or 2 is considered to represent complete metabolic response at interim and end of treatment.
- More recent data also suggest that most patients with uptake higher than mediastinum but less than or equivalent to liver (score of 3) have good prognosis at the end of treatment with standard therapy in HL [131].
- However, in response-adapted trials exploring treatment de-escalation, a more cautious approach may be preferred, judging a score of 3 to be an inadequate response to avoid undertreatment. Therefore, interpretation of a score of 3 depends on the timing of assessment, the clinical context, and the treatment.
- A score of 4 or 5 at interim suggests chemotherapy-sensitive disease, provided uptake has reduced from baseline, and is considered to represent partial metabolic response.
- A residual metabolic activity at the end of treatment with a score of 4 or 5 represents treatment failure even if uptake has reduced from baseline.
- A score of 4 or 5 with intensity that does not change or even increases from baseline and/or new foci compatible with lymphoma represents treatment failure, both at interim and at the end-of-treatment assessment.

All the above recommendations should be based on a PET scan interpretation by visual assessment. In the literature, some data suggest that a quantitative cut-off based on SUV measurement may also be interesting. For example, a recent publication [134] showed that, in a cohort of 59 HL patients treated with 4–8 cycles of anthracycline-based chemotherapy, the PET-2-positive predictive value was better using ΔSUVmax (with a cut-off of 70%) than the 5-point scale (46%). However, at the moment, there is insufficient evidence to precisely settle the adequate reduction ("delta") in FDG uptake that predicts treatment response; moreover, this quantitative phenomenon depends on the timing and intensity of the given treatment; finally, caution should be used in assessing data arising from quantitative PET scan interpretation, especially if retrospectively generated, in the absence of a defined program for PET scanner calibration, image generation, acquisition and reconstruction. Recent data also suggest that morphological information with CT evaluation may help in patients with a positive interim PET; a greater reduction in tumour size correlates with an improved outcome; for example, in 88 HL doxorubicin, vinblastine and gemcitabine (AVG)-treated patients, interim PET predicted PFS better than percent decrease in the sum of the products of the perpendicular diameters (%SPPD), but in a combined CT and PET/CT analysis, the predictive value on PFS was higher than with either test alone [135]. On the other hand, a classical anatomical CT-based response assessment is preferred for lymphoma subsets with a variable/low FDG avidity. In summary, the following recommendations have been set for end-of-treatment response assessment (Table 3.3):

1. "PET-CT should be used for response assessment in FDG-avid lymphoma, using the 5-point scale; CT is preferred for low or variable FDG avidity.
2. A complete metabolic response (CMR) even with a persistent mass is considered a complete remission.
3. A partial response by CT criteria only requires a decrease by more than 50% in the sum of the product of the perpendicular diameters of up to six representative nodes or extranodal lesions.
4. Progressive disease by CT criteria only requires an increase in the cross product of the longest transverse diameter of a lesion and perpendicular diameter of a single node by $\geq$50%.
5. Surveillance PET scans for patients in complete remission are discouraged, especially

for DLBCL and HL, although a repeat study may be considered after an equivocal finding after treatment.

6. Judicious use of follow-up scans may be considered in indolent lymphomas with residual intra-abdominal or retro-peritoneal disease."

3.8 Practical Examples on Interim and End-of Treatment PET Scan Interpretation

Case 1

G. L., female, 26 years. Since December 2008 she complained 4-limb and trunk itching and night sweats; 2 months later a supraclavicular right enlarged lymph node was palpable. Upon surgical resection the pathology examination of an enlarged left lateral cervical node revealed classic Hodgkin lymphoma, nodular sclerosis subtype. Baseline biochemical test and haemogram with complete blood count revealed a normal total and fractional leucocyte number, mild anaemia, ESR 66, and LDH 435 U/l. Viral serology was negative. Bone marrow trephine biopsy excluded the presence of lymphoma. Pregnancy test was negative.

The Staging PET/CT, performed in May 2009 (Shown in Fig. 3.9)

Left side cervical enlarged nodes were recorded, with SUVmax between 3.3 and 4.8 and in the left supraclavicular region with a SUVmax of 3.3. Another enlarged lymph node was noted in the infra-pectoral region with a SUVmax of 2.7 and a focal FDG uptake was also recorded in the left upper lung lobe corresponding to a CT-recorded opacity of 1.5 cm, with a SUVmax of 11.4. Presence of pathologically enlarged lymph nodes and partially confluent in right para-tracheal region and right pre-carinal and Barety lodge (SUVmax 9). There were no abnormal findings in the anatomical regions below the diaphragm. A diffuse pattern of FDG uptake at the skeletal bone marrow was compatible with diffuse marrow activation in the absence of focal elements.

Final Diagnosis: Classical Hodgkin Lymphoma, Nodular Sclerosis Subtype, Stage IV A (Lung)
IPS 1

The patient was enrolled in the HD0607 trial and treated with two ABVD courses from June to August 2009.

Interim PET/CT in August 2009

No evidence of pathological FDG uptake. An unspecific uptake was recorded in the tonsillar region. Upon blinded independent central review, the interim PET (PET-2) was reported as negative and the patient continued therapy with ABVD. A final evaluation by PET/CT in December 2009 (Fig. 3.10) showed complete disappearance of abnormal FDG uptake, compatible with complete metabolic response.

Case 2

B. A., female, 59 years. Since May 2010 she noted the appearance of a persistent cough, fever 38.5 °C, weight loss of about 7 kg and generalized itching. An ultrasound examination of the neck showed evidence of enlarged lymph nodes of diameter of 7 and 10 mm in the supra-clavicular and cervical right regions. In July 2010 a chest X-ray showed a mediastinal lymph node enlargement at the level of azygos vein confluence. In mid-September, a clinical examination revealed voluminous enlarged nodes in the right axilla with the largest diameter of about 5 cm and in cervical right region of about 3 cm. The baseline complete haemogram showed mild anaemia and leucocytosis. Routine biochemical blood tests were normal. A biopsy of the right cervical node showed a histological diagnosis of HL classic, nodular sclerosis subtype.

The Baseline PET, Performed in Late September 2010 (Shown in Fig. 3.11)

There was evidence of right cervical nodes with a diameter ranging from 2 to <1 cm with a SUVmax between 6.6 and 17.6. Confluent left supraclavicular lymph nodes with a SUVmax of and right confluent axillary nodal mass were recorded, with the largest diameter of 5 cm and SUVmax 12.8. A mediastinal bulky mass was also detected, with the contribution of anterior mediastinal, internal mammary and para-tracheal

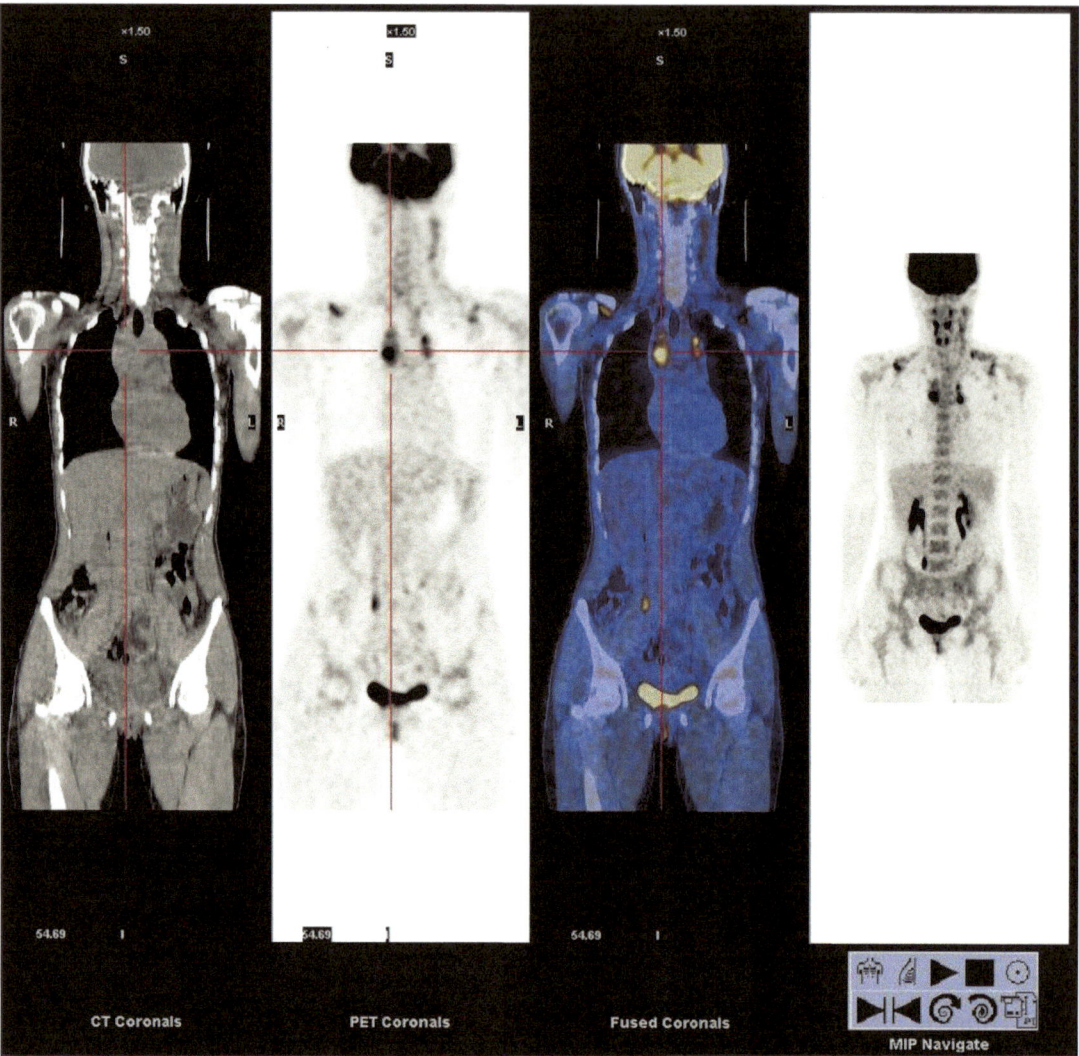

Fig. 3.10 PET/CT for staging

lymph nodes, with a SUVmax of 15.7. A pericardial effusion was present, with a SUVmax of 8.4. Several pathologically enlarged para-aortic lymph nodes, extending from D12 to L3, were also noted, showing a SUVmax of 13.6. There were no abnormal findings in the liver. The spleen was massively and focally infiltrated by lymphoma with a pathological area with the largest diameter of 9 cm and SUVmax of 13.5. There were no skeletal abnormalities.

The Final Diagnosis: Hodgkin Lymphoma, Classical, Nodular Sclerosis Subtype, Stage IIIB. IPS 2

The patient was enrolled in the HD0607 clinical trial. After 2 ABVD courses, an interim PET (PET-2) was performed, with the following local

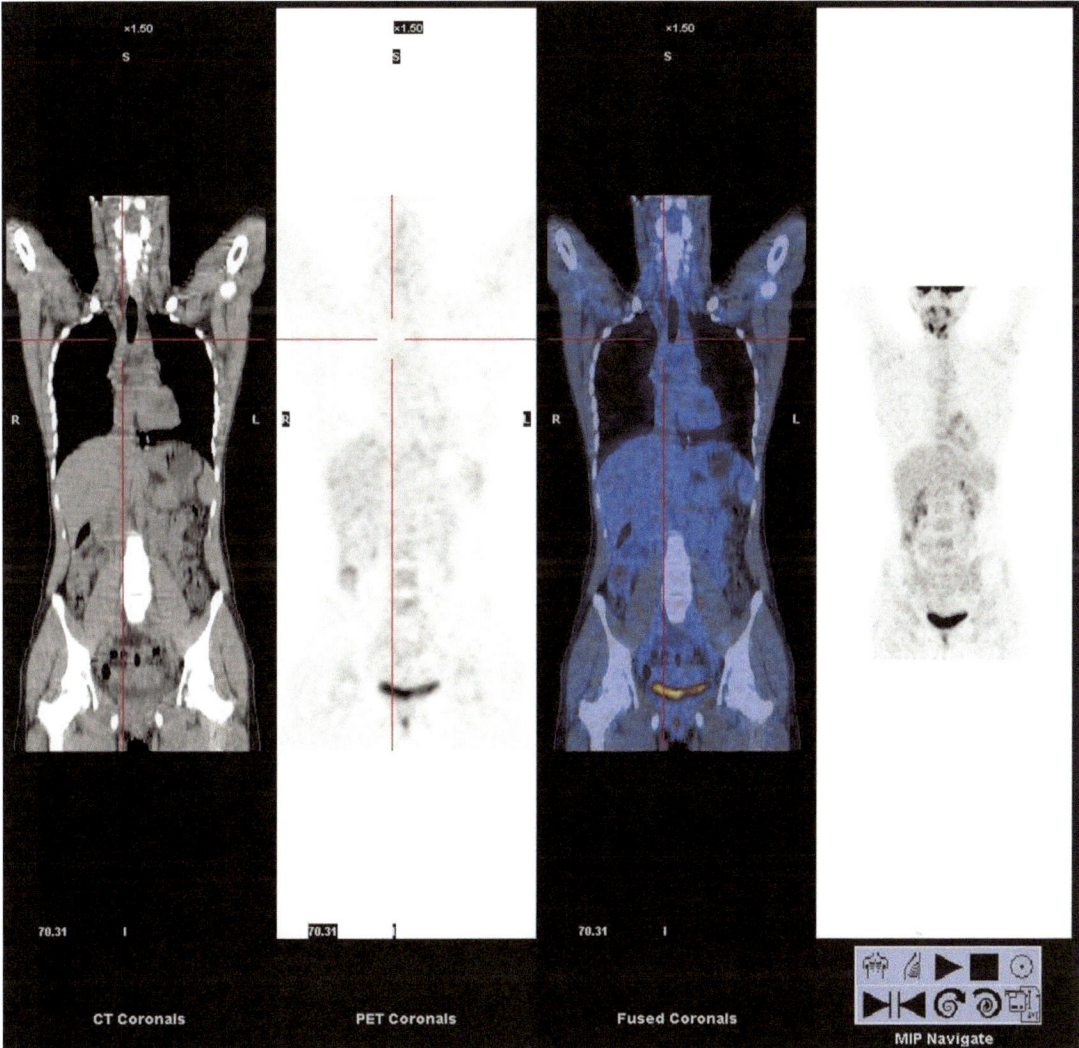

Fig. 3.11 PET/CT for interim restaging

report: probable persistence of disease in Barety lodge. There were no other sites of disease (Fig. 3.12). Upon central review PET-2 was considered positive, with a Deauville score 4 and, accordingly, the treatment was intensified with BEACOPP escalated in December 2010: two cycles were administered at full dosage and the other two with an attenuated dose (BEACOPP baseline) for neurological toxicity (WHO grade 3 peripheral neuropathy). Treatment response was assessed with PET/CT in June 2011, with evidence of complete metabolic response (CMR). The patient skipped the subsequent treatment as planned in the HD 0607 trial, for grade 3 SAE (pneumonia, occurring after the 4th cycle). The complete restaging with FDG-CT/PET in November 2011 showed CMR, and since then the patient is in continuous complete remission.

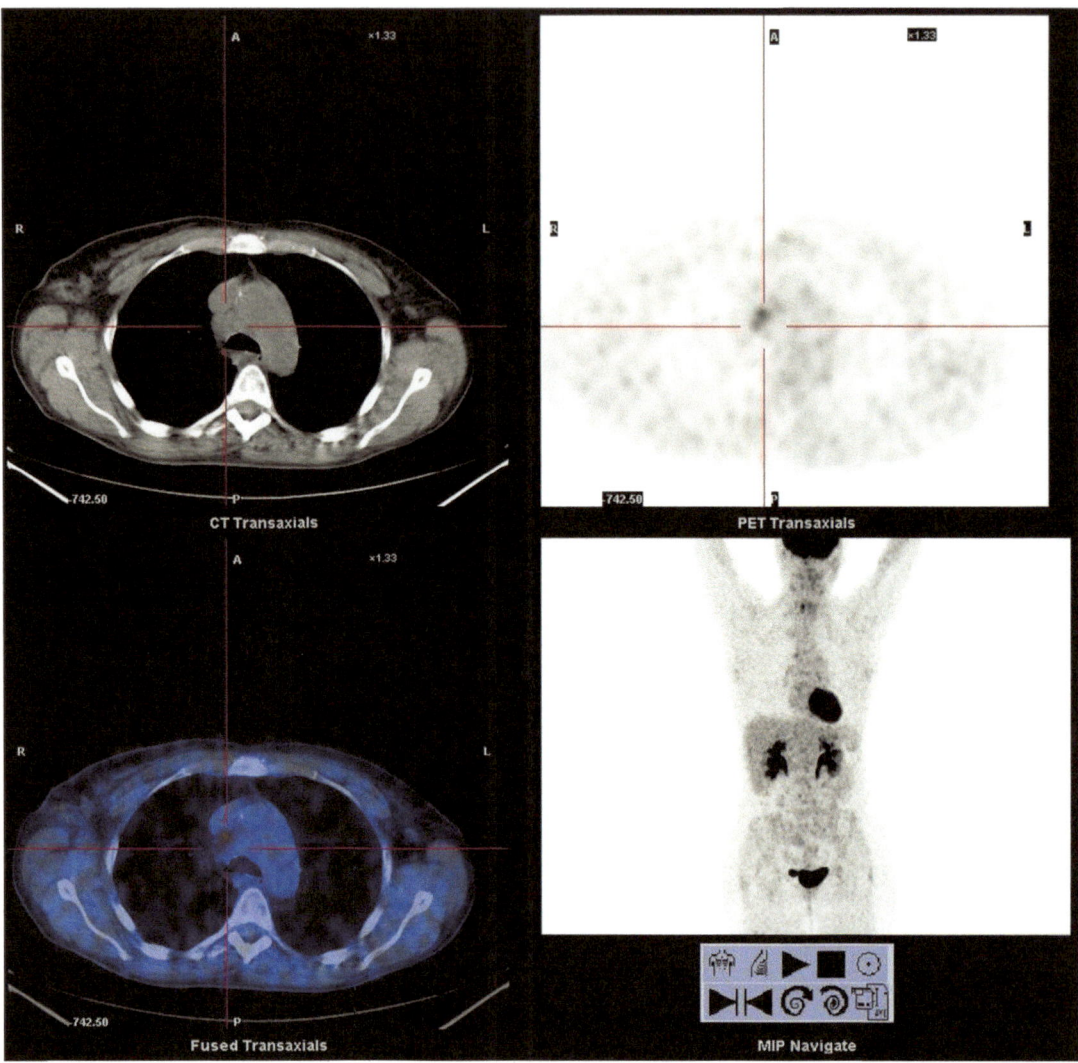

Fig. 3.12 PET/CT for end-of-treatment restaging

References

1. Kyle SD, Law WP, Miles KA. Predicting tumour response. Cancer Imaging. 2013;13(3):381–90.
2. Keepers YP, Pizao PE, Peters GJ, Van Ark-Otte J, Winograd B, Pinedo HM. Comparison of the sulforhodamine B protein and tetrazolium (MTT) assays for in vitro chemosensitivity testing. Eur J Cancer. 1991;27:897–900.
3. Unger FT, Witte I, David KA. Prediction of individual response to anticancer therapy: historical and future perspectives. Cell Mol Life Sci. 2015;72:729–57.
4. Levis A, Vitolo U, Ciocca Vasino MA, Cametti G, Urgesi A, Bertini M, et al. Predictive value of the early response to chemotherapy in high-risk stages II and III Hodgkin's disease. Cancer. 1987;60(8):1713–9.
5. Naumann R, Vaic A, Beuthien-Baumann B, Bredow J, Kropp J, Kittner T, et al. Prognostic value of positron emission tomography in the evaluation of posttreatment residual mass in patients with Hodgkin's disease and non-Hodgkin's lymphoma. Br J Haematol. 2001;115(4):793–800.
6. Radford JA, Cowan RA, Flanagan M, Durn G, Crowther D, Johnson RJ, et al. The significance of residual mediastinal abnormality on the chest radiograph following treatment for Hodgkin's disease. J Clin Oncol. 1988;6(6):940–6.
7. Weber WA. Assessing tumor response to therapy. J Nucl Med. 2009;50:1S–0.
8. Gallamini A, Hutchings M, Rigacci L, et al. Early interim 2-[18F]fluoro-2- deoxy-D glucose positron emission tomography is prognostically superior to international prognostic score in advanced-stage

Hodgkin's lymphoma: a report from a joint Italian-Danish study. J Clin Oncol. 2007;25:3746–52.

9. Lin C, Itti E, Haioun C, Petegnief Y, Luciani A, Dupuis J, et al. Early 18F-FDG PET for prediction of prognosis in patients with diffuse large B-cell lymphoma: SUV-based assessment versus visual analysis. J Nucl Med. 2007;48:1626–32.

10. Gavid M, Prevot-Bitot N, Timoschenko A, Gallet P, Martin C, Prades JM. [18F]-FDG PET-CT prediction of response to induction chemotherapy in head and neck squamous cell carcinoma: preliminary findings. Eur Ann Otorhinolaryngol Head Neck Dis. 2015;132(1):3–7.

11.; Groheux D, Sanna A, Majdoub M, de Cremoux P, Giacchetti S, Teixeira L, et al. Baseline tumour 18FDG uptake and modifications after 2 cycles of neoadjuvant chemotherapy are prognostic of outcome in ER+/HER2- breast cancer. J Nucl Med. 2015;56(6):824–31. pli: jnumed 115.154138.

12. Liu FY, Yen TC, Wang JY, Tang TS. Early prediction by 18F-FDG PET/CT for progression free survival and overall survival in patients with metastatic colorectal cancer receiving third-line cetuximab-based therapy. Clin Nucl Med. 2015;40(3):200–5.

13. Lamanna N, Jurcic JG, Noy A, Maslak P, Gencarelli AN, Panageas KS, et al. Sequential therapy with fludarabine, high-dose cyclophosphamide, and rituximab in previously untreated patients with chronic lymphocytic leukemia produces high-quality responses: molecular remissions predict for durable complete responses. J Clin Oncol. 2009;27(4):491–7.

14. Strati P, Keating MJ, O'Brien SM, Burger J, Ferrajoli A, Jain N, et al. Eradication of bone marrow minimal residual disease may prompt early treatment discontinuation in CLL. Blood. 2014;123(24):3727–32.

15. Mahon FX, Etienne G. Deep molecular response in chronic myeloid leukemia: the new goal of therapy? Clin Cancer Res. 2014;20(2):310–22.

16. Ladetto M, Lobetti-Bodoni C, Mantoan B, Ceccarelli M, Boccomini C, Genuardi E, et al. Persistence of minimal residual disease in bone marrow predicts outcome in follicular lymphomas treated with a rituximab-intensive program. Blood. 2013;122(23):3759–66.

17. Gallamini A, Kostakoglu L. Interim FDG-PET in Hodgkin lymphoma: a compass for a safe navigation in clinical trials? Blood. 2012;120(25):4913–20.

18. Carbone PP, Kaplan HS, Musshoff K, et al. Report of the committee on Hodgkin's disease staging classification. Cancer Res. 1971;31:1860–1.

19. Lister TA, Crowther D, Sutcliffe SB, Glatstein E, Canellos GP, Young RC, et al. Report of a committee convened to discuss the evaluation and staging of patients with Hodgkin disease: Cotswolds meeting. J Clin Oncol. 1989;7(11):1630–6.

20. Kaplan HS. Contiguity and progression in Hodgkin's disease. Cancer Res. 1971;31:1811–3.

21. Castellino RA, Hoppe RT, Blank N, Young SW, Neumann C, Rosenberg SA, et al. Computed tomography, lymphography, and staging laparotomy: correlations in initial staging of Hodgkin disease. AJR Am J Roentgenol. 1984;143(7):37–41.

22. Gospadorowitz MK, O'Sullivan B, Koh ES. Prognostic factors: principles and applications. In: Prognostic factors in cancer. 3rd ed. Hoboken: Wiley-Liss; 2006. p. 23–8.

23. Specht L, Hasenclever D. Prognostic factors. In: Engert A, Younes A, editors. Hodgkin lymphoma. 2nd ed. Springer; 2015. p. 131–55.

24. Gobbi PG, Ghirardelli ML, Solcia M, Di Giulio G, Merli F, Tavecchia L, et al. Image-aided estimate of tumor burden in Hodgkin's disease: evidence of its primary prognostic importance. J Clin Oncol. 2001;19:1388–94.

25. Horwich A, Easton D, Nogueira-Costa R, Liew KH, Colman M, Peckam MJ. An analysis of prognostic factors in early stage Hodgkin's disease. Radiother Oncol. 1986;7:95–106.

26. Mauch P, Tarbell N, Weinstein H, Silver B, Goffman T, Osteen R, et al. Stage IA and IIA supradiaphragmatic Hodgkin's disease: prognostic factors in surgically staged patients treated with mantle and paraaortic irradiation. J Clin Oncol. 1988;6:1576–83.

27. Gobbi PG, Broglia C, Di Giulio G, Mantelli M, Anselmo P, Merli F, et al. The clinical value of tumor burden at diagnosis in Hodgkin lymphoma. Cancer. 2004;101:1824–34.

28. Bartlett NC: Limited-stage Hodgkin lymphoma: optimal chemotherapy and the role of radiotherapy Am Soc Clin Oncol Educ Book 2013; 374-80.

29. Hasenclever D, Diehl V. A prognostic score for advanced Hodgkin's disease. N Engl J Med. 1998;339:1506–14.

30. Gobbi PG, Zinzani PL, Broglia C, Comelli M, Magagnoli M, Federico M, et al. Comparison of prognostic models in patients with advanced Hodgkin disease. Promising results from integration of the best three systems. Cancer. 2001;91:1467–78.

31. Moccia AA, Donaldson J, Chhanabhai M, Hoskins PJ, Klasa RJ, Savage KJ, et al. International prognostic score in advanced-stage Hodgkin's lymphoma: altered utility in the modern era. J Clin Oncol. 2012;30:3383–8.

32. Hutchings M, Loft A, Hansen M, Pedersen LM, Berthelsen AK, Keiding S, et al. Position emission tomography with or without computed tomography in the primary staging of Hodgkin's lymphoma. Haematologica. 2006;91:482–9.

33. Gallamini A. Positron emission tomography scanning: a new paradigm for the management of Hodgkin's lymphoma. Haematologica. 2010;95(7):1046–8.

34. Steidl C, Connors JM, Gascoyne RD. Molecular pathogenesis of Hodgkin's lymphoma: increasing evidence of the importance of the microenvironment. J Clin Oncol. 2011;29(14):1812–26.

35. Ma Y, Visser L, Roelofsen H, et al. Proteomics analysis of Hodgkin lymphoma: identification of new players lymphocytes involved in the crosstalk between HRS cells and infiltrating lymphocytes. Blood. 2008;111(4):2339–46.

36. Weiler-Sagie M, Bushelev O, Epelbaum R, et al. 18F-FDG avidity in lymphoma readdressed: a study of 766 patients. J Nucl Med. 2010;51(1):25–30.

37. Hutchings M, Loft A, Hansen M, et al. FDG-PET after two cycles of chemotherapy predicts treatment failure and progression-free survival in Hodgkin lymphoma. Blood. 2006;107(1):52–9.

38. Gallamini A, Rigacci L, Merli F, et al. The predictive value of positron emission tomography scanning performed after two courses of standard therapy on treatment outcome in advanced stage Hodgkin's disease. Haematologica. 2006;91(4):475–81.

39. Weihrauch MR, Manzke O, Beyer M, et al. Elevated serum levels of CC thymus and activation-related chemokine (TARC) in primary Hodgkin's disease: potential for a prognostic factor. Cancer Res. 2005;65(13):5516–9.

40. Plattel WJ, Van den Berg A, Visser L, et al. Plasma thymus and activation-regulated chemokine as an early response marker in classical Hodgkin's lymphoma. Haematologica. 2012;97(3):410–5.

41. Rohren EM, Turkington TG, Coleman RE. Clinical applications of PET in oncology. Radiology. 2004;231(2):305–32.

42. Evens AM, Kostakoglu L. The role of FDG-PET in defining prognosis of Hodgkin lymphoma for early-stage disease. Blood. 2014;124(23):3356–64.

43. Hutchings M, Mikhaeel NG, Fields PA, Nunan T, Timothy AR. Prognostic value of interim FDGPET after two or three cycles of chemotherapy in Hodgkin lymphoma. Ann Oncol. 2005;16(7):1160–8.

44. Straus DJ, Johnson JL, LaCasce AS, Bartlet NL, Kostakoglu L, Hsi LD, et al. Doxorubicin, vinblastine, and gemcitabine (CALGB 50203) for stage I/II nonbulky Hodgkin lymphoma: pretreatment prognostic factors and interim PET. Blood. 2011;117(20):5314–20.

45. Terasawa T, Lau J, Bardet S, et al. Fluorine-18-fluorodeoxyglucose positron emission tomography for interim response assessment of advanced stage Hodgkin's lymphoma and diffuse large B-cell lymphoma: a systematic review. J Clin Oncol. 2009;27:1906–14.

46. Zinzani PL, Tani M, Fanti S, et al. Early positron emission tomography (PET) restaging: a predictive final response in Hodgkin's disease patients. Ann Oncol. 2006;17(8):1296–300.

47. Cerci JJ, Pracchia LF, Linardi CCG, Pitella FA, Delbeke D, Izaki M, et al. 18F-FDG PET after 2 cycles of ABVD predicts event-free survival in early and advanced Hodgkin Lymphoma. J Nucl Med. 2010;51:1337–43.

48. Gallamini A, Barrington SF, Biggi A, Chauvie S, Kostakoglu L, Gregianin M, et al. The predictive role of interim positron emission tomography for Hodgkin lymphoma treatment outcome is confirmed using the interpretation criteria of the Deauville five-point scale. Haematologica. 2014;99(6):1107–13.

49. Kostakoglu L, Coleman M, Leonard JP, Kuji I, Zoe H, Goldsmith SJ. PET predicts prognosis after 1 cycle of chemotherapy in aggressive lymphoma and Hodgkin's disease. J Nucl Med. 2002;43:1018–27.

50. Kostakoglu L, Goldsmith SJ, Leonard JP, Christos P, Furman RR, Atasever T, et al. FDG-PET after 1 cycle of therapy predicts outcome in diffuse large cell lymphoma and classic Hodgkin disease. Cancer. 2006;107:2678–87.

51. Hutchings M, Kostakoglu L, Zaucha JM, et al. In vivo treatment sensitivity testing with positron emission tomography/computed tomography after one cycle of chemotherapy for Hodgkin lymphoma. J Clin Oncol. 2014;32:2705–11.

52. Diehl V, Stein H, Hummel M, Zollinger R, Connors JM. Hodgkin's lymphoma: biology and treatment strategies for primary, refractory, and relapsed disease. Hematology Am Soc Hematol Educ Program. 2003(1);225–47.

53. Bonadonna G, Viviani S, Bonfante V, Gianni AM, Valagussa P. Survival in Hodgkin's disease patients – report of 25 years of experience at the Milan cancer Institute. Eur J Cancer. 2005;41(7):998–1006.

54. Armitage JO. Early-stage Hodgkin's lymphoma. N Engl J Med. 2010;363:653–62.

55. Behringer K, Breuer K, Reineke T, May M, Nogova L, Klimm B, et al. Secondary amenorrhea after Hodgkin's lymphoma is influenced by age at treatment, stage of disease, chemotherapy regimen, and the use of oral contraceptives during therapy: a report from the German Hodgkin's Lymphoma Study Group. J Clin Oncol. 2005;23:7555–64.

56. Engert A, Diehl V, Franklin J, Lohri A, Dorken B, Ludwing WD, et al. Escalated-dose BEACOPP in the treatment of patients with advanced-stage Hodgkin's lymphoma: 10 years of follow-up of the GHSG HD9 study. J Clin Oncol. 2009;27:4548–54.

57. Freedman AS, Neuberg D, Mauch P, Soiffer RJ, Anderson KC, Fisher DC, et al. Longterm follow-up of autologous bone marrow transplantation in patients with relapsed follicular lymphoma. Blood. 1999;94:3325–33.

58. Rambaldi A, Carlotti E, Oldani E, Della Starza I, Baccarani M, Cortelazzo S, et al. Quantitative PCR of bone marrow BCL2/IgH+ cells at diagnosis predicts lymphoma treatment response and long-term outcome in follicular non-Hodgkin lymphoma. Blood. 2005;105:3428–33.

59. Ziakas PD, Poulou LS. Improving outcome after positive interim PET in advanced Hodgkin's disease: reality vs. expectation. Eur J Nucl Med Mol Imaging. 2008;35(8):1573–5.

60. Kasamon Y. Prognostication and risk-adapted therapy of Hodgkin's lymphoma using positron emission tomography. Adv Hematol. 2011;271595:1–12.

61. Laskar S, Gupta T, Vimal S, et al. Consolidation radiation after complete remission in Hodgkin's disease following six cycles of doxorubicin, bleomycin, vinblastine, and dacarbazine chemotherapy: is there a need? J Clin Oncol. 2004;22(1):62–8.

62. Meyer RM, Gospodarowicz MK, Connors JM, et al. randomized comparison of ABVD chemotherapy

with a strategy that includes radiation therapy in patients with limited-stage Hodgkin's lymphoma: National Cancer Institute of Canada Clinical Trials Group and the Eastern Cooperative Oncology Group. J Clin Oncol. 2005;23(21):4634–42.

63. Nachman JB, Sposto R, Herzog P, et al. Randomized comparison of low-dose involved field radiotherapy and no radiotherapy for children with Hodgkin's disease who achieve a complete response to chemotherapy. J Clin Oncol. 2002;20(18):3765–71.

64. Straus DJ, Portlock CS, Qin J, et al. Results of a prospective randomized clinical trial of doxorubicin, bleomycin, vinblastine, and dacarbazine (ABVD) followed by radiation therapy (RT) versus ABVD alone for stages I, II, and IIIA nonbulky Hodgkin disease. Blood. 2004;104(12):3483–9.

65. Meyer RM, Gospodarowicz MK, Connors JM, et al. ABVD alone versus radiation-based therapy in limited-stage Hodgkin's lymphoma. N Engl J Med. 2012;366(5):399–408.

66. Hay AE, Klimm B, Chen BE, et al. An individual patient-data comparison of combined modality therapy and ABVD alone for patients with limited stage Hodgkin lymphoma. Ann Oncol. 2013;24(12):3065–9.

67. Sher DJ, Mauch PM, Van Den Abbeele A, LaCasce AS, Czerminski J, Ng AK. Prognostic significance of mid- and post-ABVD PET imaging in Hodgkin's lymphoma: the importance of involved-field radiotherapy. Ann Oncol. 2009;20:1848–53.

68. Le Roux PY, Gastinne T, Le Gouill S, Nowak E, Bodet-Milin C, Querellou S, et al. Prognostic value of interim FDG PET/CT in Hodgkin's lymphoma patients treated with interim response-adapted strategy: comparison of International Harmonization Project (IHP), Gallamini and London criteria. Eur J Nucl Med Mol Imaging. 2011;38(6):1064–71.

69. Picardi M, De Renzo A, Pane F, Nicolai E, Pacelli R, Salvatore M, et al. Randomized comparison of consolidation radiation versus observation in bulky Hodgkin's lymphoma with post-chemotherapy negative positron emission tomography scans. Leuk Lymphoma. 2007;48(9):1721–7.

70. Radford J, Illidge T, Counsell N, Hancock B, Pettengell R, Johnson P, et al. Results of a trial of PET-directed therapy for early-stage Hodgkin's lymphoma. N Engl J Med. 2015;372:1598–607.

71. Meignan M, Gallamini A, Haioun C. Report on the first international workshop on interim-PET scan in lymphoma. Leuk Lymphoma. 2009;50(8):1257–60.

72. Raemaekers JMM, André MPE, Federico M, Girinsky T, Oumedaly R, Brusamolino E, et al. Omitting radiotherapy in early Positron Emission Tomography-negative stage I/II Hodgkin Lymphoma is associated with an increased risk of early relapse: clinical results of the pre-planned interim analysis of the randomized EORTC/LYSA/FIL H10 Trial. J Clin Oncol. 2014;32(12):1188–94.

73. Raemaekers JMN, Andrè MPE, Federico M, et al. Early FDG-PET adapted treatment improves the

outcome of early FDG-PET positive patients with stage I/II Hodgkin lymphoma (HL): final results of the randomized Intergroup EORTC/LYSA/FIL H10 trial. Hematol Oncol. 2015;33(Suppl 1 June 2015):abstract 117a.

74. HD16 for early stage Hodgkin lymphoma. Clinicaltrials.gov web site. http://clinicaltrials.gov/ct2/show/NCT00736320. Accessed 31 May 2013.

75. HD17 for intermediate stage Hodgkin lymphoma. Clinicaltrials.gov web site. http://www.clinicaltrials.gov/ct2/show/NCT01356680. Accessed 31 May 2013.

76. Response-based therapy assessed by PET scan in treating patients with bulky stage I and stage II classical Hodgkin lymphoma (CALGB 50801). Clinicaltrials.gov web site. http://www.clinicaltrials.gov/ct2/show/NCT01118026. Accessed 31 May 2013.

77. Chemotherapy based on PET scan in treating patients with stage I or stage II Hodgkin lymphoma (ECOG). Clinicaltrials.gov web site. http://www.clinicaltrials.gov/ct2/show/NCT01390584. Accessed 31 May 2013.

78. Federico M, Bellei M, Cheson BD. BEACOPP or no BEACOPP? Lancet Oncol. 2013;14(12):e487–8.

79. Viviani S, Zinzani PL, Rambaldi A, et al. ABVD versus BEACOPP for Hodgkin's lymphoma when high-dose salvage is planned. N Engl J Med. 2011;365:203–12.

80. Federico M, Luminari S, Iannitto E, Polimeno G, Marcheselli L, Montanini A, et al. ABVD compared with BEACOPP, compared with CEC for the initial treatment of patients with advanced Hodgkin's lymphoma: results from the HD2000 Gruppo Italiano per lo Studio dei Linfomi Trial. J Clin Oncol. 2009;27:805–11.

81. Mounier N, Brice P, Bologna S, et al. ABVD (8 cycles) versus BEACOPP (4 escalated cycles ≥ 4 baseline): final results in stage III-IV low-risk Hodgkin lymphoma (IPS 0-2) of the LYSA H34 randomized trial. Ann Oncol. 2014;25(8):1622–8.

82. Borchmann P, Diehl V, Engert A. ABVD versus BEACOPP for Hodgkin's lymphoma. N Engl J Med. 2011;365(16):1545–6.

83. Bauer K, Skoetz N, Monsef I, et al. Comparison of chemotherapy including escalated BEACOPP versus chemotherapy including ABVD for patients with early unfavourable or advanced stage Hodgkin lymphoma. Cochrane Database Syst Rev. 2011;8:CD007941–CD007941.

84. Gallamini A, Patti C, Viviani S, Rossi A, Fiore F, Di Raimondo F, et al. Early chemotherapy intensification with BEACOPP in advanced stage Hodgkin lymphoma patients with a interim-PET positive after two ABVD courses. Br J Haematol. 2011;152(5):551–60.

85. Ganesan P, Rajendranath R, Kannan K, Radhakrishnan V, Ganesan TS, Udupa K, et al. Phase II study of Interim PET-CT guided response adapted therapy in advanced Hodgkin's lymphoma. Ann Oncol. 2015;26(6):1170–4. pii: mdv077.

86. Deau B, Franchi P, Briere J, Ohnona J, Tamburini J, Thieblemont C, Brice P. PET2-driven de-escalation therapy in 64 high-risk Hodgkin lymphoma patients treated with escalated BEACOPP. Br J Haematol. 2015. doi:10.1111/bjh.13287 [Epub ahead of print].

87. Positron emission tomography (PET)-adapted chemotherapy in advanced Hodgkin lymphoma (HL) (HD0607). Clinicaltrials.gov web site. http://www.clinicaltrials.gov/ct2/show/NCT00795613. Accessed 31 May 2013.

88. Fludeoxyglucose F 18-PET/CT imaging in assessing response to chemotherapy in patients with newly diagnosed stage II, stage III, or stage IV Hodgkin lymphoma (RATHL). Clinicaltrials.gov web site. http://www.clinicaltrials.gov/ct2/show/NCT00678327. Accessed 31 May 2013.

89. Fludeoxyglucose F 18-PET/CT imaging and combination chemotherapy with or without additional chemotherapy and G-CSF in treating patients with stage III or stage IV Hodgkin lymphoma (SWOG-CALG-B). Clinicaltrials.gov web site. http://clinicaltrials.gov/ct2/show/NCT00822120. Accessed 31 May 2013.

90. Press OW, LeBlanc M, Rimsza LM, Schoder H, Friedberg JW, Evens AM, et al. A phase II trial of response-adapted therapy of stages III-IV Hodgkin lymphoma using early interim FDG-PET imaging: US intergroup S0816. Hematol Oncol. 2013;31(Suppl 1):137. Abstract 124.

91. Johnson P, Federico M, Fossa A, O'Doherty M, Roberts T, Stevens L, et al. Response-adapted therapy based on interim FDG-PET scans in advanced Hodgkin lymphoma: first analysis of the safety of de-escalation and efficacy of escalation in the international RATHL study (CRUK/07/033). Hematol Oncol. 2015;33(Suppl 1 June 2015):102, Abstract 008.

92. Gallamini A, Rossi A, Patti C, Picardi M, Di Raimondo F, Cantonetti M, et al. Interim-PET adapted chemotherapy in advanced Hodgkin lymphoma: results of the second interim analysis of the Italian GITIL/FIL HD0607 trial. Hematol Oncol. 2015;33(Suppl 1 June 2015):163, Abstract 118.

93. Dodd LE, Korn EL, Freidlin B, Jaffe CC, Rubinstein LV, Dancey J, et al. Blinded independent central review of progression-free survival in phase III clinical trials: important design element or unnecessary expense? Clin Oncol. 2008;26:3791–6.

94. Amit O, Bushnell W, Dodd L, Roach N, Sargent D. Blinded independent central review of the progression-free survival endpoint. Oncologist. 2010;15:492–5.

95. Chauvie S, Biggi A, Stancu A, Cerello P, Cavallo A, Fallanca F, et al. WIDEN: a tool for medical image management in multicentre clinical trials. Clin Trials. 2014;11:355–61.

96. Tailored therapy for Hodgkin lymphoma using early interim therapy PET for therapy decision. Clinicaltrials.gov web site. http://www.clinicaltrials.gov/ct2/show/NCT00392314. Accessed 31 May 2013.

97. Dann EJ, Bairey O, Bar-Shalom R, Izak M, Koremberg A, Akria L, et al. Tailored therapy in Hodgkin lymphoma, based on predefined risk factors and early interim PET/CT, Israeli H2 protocol: preliminary report on 317 patients. Haematologica. 2013;98(Suppl 2):37. Abstract T110.

98. Brucher BL, Weber W, Bauer M, Fink U, Avril N, Stein HJ, Werner M, Zimmerman F, Siewert JR, Schwaiger M. Neoadjuvant therapy of esophageal squamous cell carcinoma: response evaluation by positron emission tomography. Ann Surg. 2001;233:300–9.

99. Vansteenkiste JF, Stroobants SG, de Leyn PR, Dupont PJ, Verbeken EK. Potentialuse of FDG-PET scan after induction chemotherapy in surgically staged IIIa-N2 non-small-cell lung cancer: a prospective pilot study. The Leuven Lung Cancer Group. Ann Oncol. 1998;9:1193–8.

100. Canellos GP. Residual mass in lymphoma may not be residual disease. J Clin Oncol. 1988;6(6):931–3.

101. Porceddu SV, Pryor DI, Burmeister E, Burmeister BH, Poulsen MG, Foote MC, Panizza B, Coman S, McFarlane D, Coman W, et al. Results of a prospective study of positron emission tomography-directed management of residual nodal abnormalities innodepositive head and neck cancer after definitive radiotherapy with or without systemic therapy. Head Neck. 2011;33:1675–82.

102. Van den Abbeele AD. The lessons of GIST—PET and PET/CT: a New paradigm for imaging. Oncologist. 2008;13:8–13.

103. Terasawa T, Nihashi T, Hotta T, Nagai H. 18F-FDG PET for post therapy assessment of Hodgkin's disease and aggressive Non-Hodgkin's lymphoma: a systematic review. J Nucl Med. 2008;49(1):13–21.

104. Engert A, Haverkamp H, Kobe C, Markova J, Renner C, Ho A, et al. Reduced-intensity chemotherapy and PET-guided radiotherapy in patients with advanced stage Hodgkin's lymphoma (HD15 trial): a randomised, open-label, phase 3 noninferiority trial. Lancet. 2012;379(9828):1791–9.

105. Magagnoli M, Marzo K, Balzarotti M, Rodari M, Mazza R, Giordano L, et al. Dimension of residual CT scan mass in Hodgkin's lymphoma (HL) is a negative prognostic factor in patients with PET negative after chemo+/– radiotherapy. Blood. 2011;118:Abstract 93.

106. Kobe C, Kuhnert G, Kahraman D, Haverkamp H, Eich HT, Franke M, et al. Assessment of tumor size reduction improves outcome prediction of Positron Emission Tomography/Computed Tomography after chemotherapy in advanced stage Hodgkin lymphoma. J Clin Oncol. 2014;32:1776–81.

107. Savage KJ, Connors JM, Klasa RJ, et al. The use of FDG-PET to guide consolidative radiotherapy in patients with advanced stage Hodgkin lymphoma with residual abnormalities on CT scan following ABVD chemotherapy [abstract]. J Clin Oncol. 2011;29(15 Suppl):8034.

108. Spaepen K, Stroobants S, Dupont P, et al. [(18)F] FDG PET monitoring of tumour response tochemotherapy: does [(18)F]FDG uptake correlate with the

viable tumour cell fraction? Eur J Nucl Med Mol Imaging. 2003;30:682–8.

109. Brice P, Bouabdallah R, Moreau P, et al. Prognostic factors for survival after high-dose therapy and autologous stem cell transplantation for patients with relapsing Hodgkin's disease: analysis of 280 patients from the French registry. Société Française de Greffe de Moëlle. Bone Marrow Transplant. 1997;20:21–6.

110. Josting A, Muller H, Borchmann P, Baars JW, Metzner B, Dohner H, et al. Dose intensity of chemotherapy in patients with relapsed Hodgkin's Lymphoma. J Clin Oncol. 2010;28:5074–80.

111. Moskowitz AJ, Yahalom J, Kewalramani T, et al. Pre-transplantation functional imaging predicts outcome following autologous stem cell transplantation for relapsed and refractory Hodgkin lymphoma. Blood. 2010;116:4934–7.

112. Moskowitz CH, Matasar MJ, Zelenetz AD, et al. Normalization of pre-ASCT, FDG-PET imaging with second line, non-cross-resistant, chemotherapy programs improves event-free survival in patients with Hodgkin lymphoma. Blood. 2012;119: 1665–70.

113. Poulou LS, Thanos L, Ziakas PD. Unifying the predictive value of pre-transplant FDG PET in patients with lymphoma: a review and meta-analysis of published trials. Eur J Nucl Med Mol Imaging. 2010;37:156–62.

114. Gentzler RD, Evens AM, Rademaker AW, Weitner BB, Mittal BB, Dillehay GL, et al. F-18 FDG-PET predicts outcomes for patients receiving total lymphoid irradiation and autologous blood stem-cell transplantation for relapsed and refractory Hodgkin lymphoma. Br J Haematol. 2014;165:793–800.

115. Moskowitz AJ, Schöder H, Yahalom J, McCall SJ, Fox SY, Gerecitano J, et al. PET-adapted sequential salvage therapy with brentuximab vedotin followed by augmented Ifosfamide, carboplatin, and etoposide for patients with relapsed and refractory Hodgkin's lymphoma: a non-randomised, open-label, single-centre, phase 2 study. Lancet Oncol. 2015;16(3):284–92.

116. Barrington SF, Mikhaeel NG, Kostakoglu L, Meignan M, Hutchings M, Müeller SP, et al. Role of imaging in the staging and response assessment of lymphoma: consensus of the International Conference on Malignant Lymphomas Imaging Working Group. J Clin Oncol. 2014;32(27): 3048–58.

117. Castagna L, Bramanti S, Balzarotti M, Sarina B, Todisco E, Anastasia A, et al. Predictive value of early 18F-fluorodeoxyglucose positron emission tomography (FDG-PET) during salvage chemotherapy in relapsing/refractory Hodgkin Lymphoma (HL) treated with high-dose chemotherapy. Br J Haematol. 2009;145:369–72.

118. Younes A, et al. Brentuximab vedotin (SGN-35) for relapsed CD30-positive lymphomas. N Engl J Med. 2010;363(19):1812–21.

119. Younes A, Gopal AK, Smith SE, Ansell SM, Rosenblatt JD, Savage KJ, et al. Results of a pivotal phase II study of Brentuximab Vedotin for patients with relapsed or refractory Hodgkin's Lymphoma. J Clin Oncol. 2012;30:2183–9.

120. Kahraman D, Theurich S, Rothe A, Kuhnert G, Sasse S, Scheid C, et al. 18-Fluorodeoxyglucose positron emission tomography/computed tomography for assessment of response to brentuximab vedotin treatment in relapsed and refractory Hodgkin lymphoma. Leuk Lymphoma. 2014;55(4):811–6.

121. Juweid ME, Stroobants S, Hoekstra OS, Mottaghy FM, Dietlein M, Guermazi A, et al. Use of positron emission tomography for response assessment of lymphoma: consensus of the Imaging Subcommittee of International Harmonization Project in Lymphoma. J Clin Oncol Off J Am Soc Clin Oncol. 2007; 25(5):571–8.

122. Zinzani PL, Viviani S, Anastasia A, Vitolo U, Luminari S, Zaja F, et al. Brentuximab vedotin in relapsed/refractory Hodgkin's lymphoma: the Italian experience and results of its use in daily clinical practice outside clinical trials. Haematologica. 2013;98(8):1232–6.

123. Cheson BD, Horning SJ, Coiffier B, Shipp MA, Fisher RI, Connors JM, et al. Report of an international workshop to standardize response criteria for non-Hodgkin's lymphomas. NCI Sponsored International Working Group. J Clin Oncol 1999; 17(4):1244–1257.

124. Cheson BD, Pfistner B, Juweid ME, Gascoyne RD, Specht L, Horning SJ, et al. Revised response criteria for malignant lymphoma. J Clin Oncol Off J Am Soc Clin Oncol. 2007;25(5):579–86.

125. Meignan M, Gallamini A, Itti E, Barrington S, Haioun C, Polliack A. Report on the third international workshop on interim positron emission tomography in lymphoma held in Menton, France, 26–27 September 2011 and Menton 2011 consensus. Leuk Lymphoma. 2012;53(10):1876–81.

126. Meignan M, Barrington S, Itti E, Gallamini A, Haioun C, Polliack A. Report on the 4th international workshop on positron emission tomography in lymphoma held in Menton, France, 3–5 October 2012. Leuk Lymphoma. 2014;55(1):31–7.

127. Wahl RL, Jacene H, Kasamon Y, Lodge MA. From RECIST to PERCIST: evolving considerations for PET response criteria in solid tumors. J Nucl. Med. 2009;50(5):122S–150S.

128. Gallamini A, Fiore F, Sorasio R, Meignan M. Interim positron emission tomography scan in Hodgkin lymphoma: definitions, interpretation rules, and clinical validation. Leuk Lymphoma. 2009;50(11):1761–4.

129. Barrington SF, Qian W, Somer EJ, Franceschetto A, Bagni B, Brun E, et al. Concordance between four European centres of PET reporting criteria designed for use in multicentre trials in Hodgkin lymphoma. Eur J Nucl Med Mol Imaging. 2010;37(10):1824–33.

130. Meignan M, Gallamini A, Haioun C, Polliack A. Report on the second international workshop on interim positron emission tomography in lymphoma held in Menton, France, 8-9 April 2010. Leuk Lymphoma. 2010;51(12):2171–80.

131. Biggi A, Gallamini A, Chauvie S, Hutchings M, Kostakoglu L, Gregianin M, et al. International validation study for interim PET in ABVD-treated, advanced-stage Hodgkin lymphoma: interpretation criteria and concordance rate among reviewers. J Nucl Med Off Publ Soc Nucl Med. 2013;54(5):683–90.

132. Meignan M, Gallamini A, Haioun C, Barrington S, Itti E, Luminari S, et al. Report on the 5 international workshop on positron emission tomography in lymphoma held in Menton, France, 19–20 September 2014. Leuk Lymphoma 2015; 56(5):1229–32.

133. Cheson BD, Fisher RI, Barrington SF, Cavalli F, Schwartz LH, Zucca E, et al. Recommendations for initial evaluation, staging, and response assessment of Hodgkin and non-Hodgkin lymphoma: the Lugano classification. J Clin Oncol Off J Am Soc Clin Oncol. 2014;32(27):3059–68.

134. Rossi C, Kanoun S, Berriolo-Riedinger A, Dygai-Cochet I, Humbert O, Legouge C, et al. Interim 18F-FDG PET SUVmax reduction is superior to visual analysis in predicting outcome early in Hodgkin lymphoma patients. J Nucl Med Off Publ Soc Nucl Med. 2014;55(4):569–73.

135. Kostakoglu L, Schoder H, Johnson JL, Hall NC, Schwartz LH, Straus DJ, et al. Interim [(18)F]fluoro-deoxyglucose positron emission tomography imaging in stage. Leuk Lymphoma. 2012;53(11):2143–50.

Lale Kostakoglu and Stephane Chauvie

4.1 Methodological Considerations

4.1.1 PET-Derived Quantitative Metrics

4.1.1.1 Standardized Uptake Value (SUV)

SUV is the most frequently used semiquantitative PET metric for measuring tumor glucose metabolism. It is defined as the ratio of the decay corrected FDG concentration in a volume of interest (VOI) to the injected dose normalized to the patient's body weight. Besides body weight-based SUV, various other SUVs have been introduced to account for the different bio-distribution of FDG in different body compositions (Table 4.1). The most commonly used is SUL, which is SUV corrected per the lean body mass (LBM) defined, respectively, for male and female as

$$LBM = 1.1 \times weight - 120 \times (weight / height)^2$$
$$LBM = 1.07 \times weight - 148 \times (weight / height)^2$$

This index takes into account the different bio-distribution of FDG in the fat tissue. Even if several recommendations exist to use SUL, e.g., in the treatment response evaluation [4], actually it is not of widespread use because of the familiarity established with SUVmax. The general advice, also furnished by the EANM-SNM guidelines on FDG-PET use [1, 3], is to collect SUL along with SUV data to further the understanding of its relevance to in both clinical practice and experimental settings. The SUV, being an index of PET tracer uptake in any tissue should be measured in a known volume of interest (VOI), because with different VOIs its measure considerably varies.

SUV_{max} The SUV_{max} is defined as the maximum value for SUV in a VOI. The rationale is choosing the single point that represents the hottest uptake or highest metabolism in the tumor. This rationale is quite strong and moreover the SUV_{max} is simple to measure. However, being a single voxel measurement, SUV_{max} is intrinsically vulnerable to image noise (Fig. 4.1). Consequently, repeated tumor SUV_{max} measurements showed an intra-patient bias of 5–30 % [5].

SUV_{mean} The SUV_{mean} is the average value of different measurements of SUVs within the VOI drawn for the tumor. It is much less vulnerable to

L. Kostakoglu, MD, MPH (✉)
Nuclear Medicine and Molecular Imaging,
Department of Radiology, Icahn School of Medicine at Mount Sinai, One Gustave L. Levy Place, Box 1141, New York, NY 10029, USA
e-mail: Lale.kostakoglu@mssm.edu

S. Chauvie
Department of Medical Physics, 'Santa Croce e Carle' Hospital, Cuneo, Italy

© Springer International Publishing Switzerland 2016
A. Gallamini (ed.), *PET Scan in Hodgkin Lymphoma*, DOI 10.1007/978-3-319-31797-7_4

Table 4.1 Pros and cons of different SUV measures

	SUV_{max}	SUV_{peak}	SUV_{mean}	MTV	TGV
Volume of interest (VOI)	Single point	1 cm³	Variable	Variable	Variable
Number of voxels in VOI	1	10–30	Hundreds–thousands	Hundreds–thousands	Hundreds–thousands
Intra-patient repeatability	5–30% [4]	1–11% [4]	Depends on segmentation method	Depends on segmentation method	Depends on segmentation method
Affected by image noise	Strongly	Slightly	Moderately	Slightly	Slightly

image noise, but it heavily depends on the delineation method used for drawing the VOI and the selected region within the tumor volume [6]. Defining a VOI in a tumor mass may have different meanings depending on its coverage within the mass. Generally one would like to provide SUV_{mean} of the entire lesion but this requires the knowledge of the exact dimension and borders with respect to the background, but this is often not the case in routine applications. An alternative approach includes delineation of a VOI inside the tumor far from its border to minimize the effect of the background uptake on the SUV measurement. Nonetheless, VOI delineation is subjective; tumors are usually heterogeneous and/or sometimes associated with necrotic centers; finally, the rationale for selecting only a part of the tumor without including the hottest part defeats the purpose of obtaining an accurate measurement.

SUV_{peak} The SUV_{peak} represents the maximum tumor activity within a 1 cm³ VOI in the hottest part of the tumor volume [3, 6]. The rationale is to have an index measurement associated with the hottest part of the tumor, i.e., SUV_{max}, but in a standard volume of 1 cm³. The SUV_{peak} characteristically is less affected by the noise compared to SUV_{max} and does not require definition of tumor boundaries which is a necessary step for obtaining an SUV_{mean}. Repeat tumor SUV_{peak} measurements yields a lower within-patient bias (1–11%) compared to those of SUV_{max} [5]. The SUV_{peak} is the proposed measurement in the definition of therapy response for PET response criteria in solid tumors (PERCIST) developed by Wahl

et al. [4]. Nonetheless, despite being relatively simple, this method requires the careful use of custom software on a dedicated workstation to be accurately calculated.

4.1.1.2 Sources of Errors in SUV Measurements

Common sources of errors involved in SUV measurements from technical and host-related factors are summarized in Table 4.2. Extensive review in literature exists to discuss these factors [1, 2], and recommendations have also been released by the US and European nuclear medicine associations [1, 3]. The recommendations provided should be considered to be minimal standards to abide by and should be followed by all imaging centers. While several recommendations are easy to adopt in clinical practice, e.g., maintaining a rest state during uptake time, others are more difficult to achieve in a busy clinic, e.g., the consistent time interval for the uptake period. Importantly, the higher the level of standardization reached, the simpler it will be to compare PET metrics acquired at different time points (intra-patient) and between different patients (inter-patient) either at a single site or across multiple centers.

Technical (Site) Factors

Several factors are patient independent and/or dependent only on the equipment and the procedure used by the site to perform PET/CT imaging studies. The requirements to limit the influence of these factors on SUV measurements should be fulfilled on one occasion and verified periodically (Table 4.2). The cross-calibration of PET scanners and activity calibrators are essential to

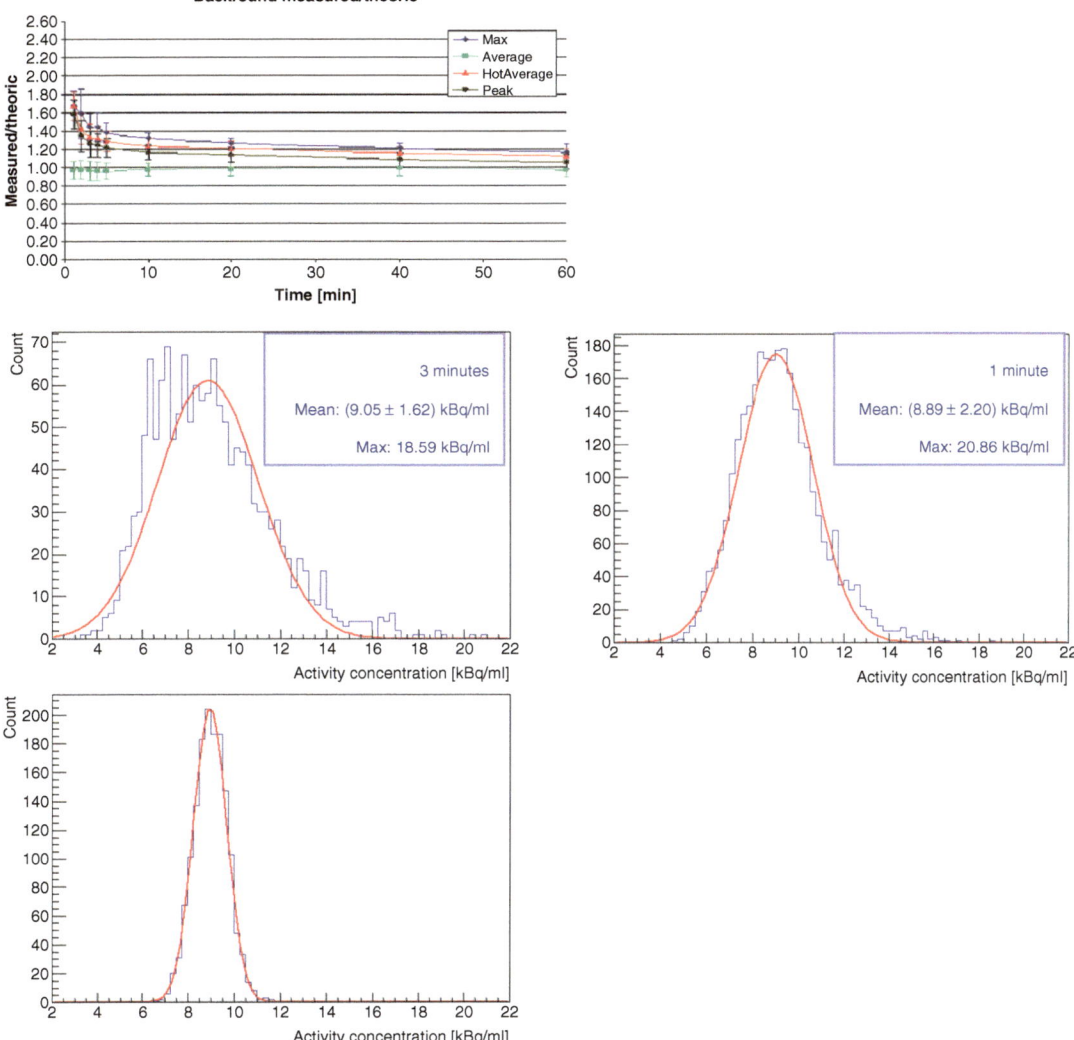

Fig. 4.1 The detailed characteristics of the noise affecting PET images are often not well known. Typically, it is assumed that overall the noise may be characterized as Gaussian. Noise levels observed in PET images complicate their interpretation; since the measurement of uniformity is strictly connected with the noise. In the figure the different metrics used for measuring activity concentration are "max," the highest pixel value; "hot," the average pixel value in a 1 cm diameter region around the "max;" "peak," the average pixel value in a 1 cm diameter ROI in the hottest region; and "average," the average of all the pixel value encompassed in the region of interest. In this figure one can see how the metrics described in the text with the acquisition time changes inside a large uniform VOI placed in the center of a uniform phantom. "Max," "hot," and "peak" have a similar trend and are the most influenced by statistics. When increasing the acquisition duration, these values decrease and the measured activity concentration become closer to the estimated values. On the other hand "average" does not change with the scan duration, and the value of the ratio between the measured and the expected activity is always about one. Errors are larger for "max," "hot," and "peak" at lower statistics, while "average" is more or less constant because its value is averaged on a large number of pixels. SUVmean is a good description of the expected value while "peak" and "max" are always overestimating the real value. And this changes dramatically when the acquisition time is small. This is well explained in the following histogram describing the SUV distribution inside the same VOI. While mean value is constant independent of the acquisition time "peak" and "max" are much larger at small time

Table 4.2 Common sources of error in SUV calculations

Source of errors	Typical errors (routine)[a]	Expected errors (controlled environment)	Action to be carried out[b]	Performed
Scanner and activity meter calibration	30%	10%	Scanner calibration: mean activity concentration in a homogenous area of phantom should be within ±3% of the expected value. Activity-meter calibration: mean activity of a radioactive source should be within ±3% of expected value	Per scanner, annually
Syringe residual	5%	0.1%	Rinsing syringe with saline is strongly recommended. Injected activity can be corrected with measured residual activity in the syringe. Alternatively a fixed value of the residual activity should be used if an evaluation of the mean activity in the syringe is carried out in the site on a statistically sufficient number of patients	Per patient
Clock time differences	10%	1%	Clock used to measure time of injected and residual activity measurements and injection and acquisition time should be synchronized (±30 s)	Per site, annually
Quality of administration	50%	0% (with patient exclusion)	An evaluation of extravasation should be carried out including the point of injection of the tracer in PET scan. For example, if intravenous injection is carried out in the harm, the patient could position the harms over the head, but the PET scan must include them in the longitudinal field of view	Per patient
Imaging parameters[c]	30%	10%	Mean recovery coefficient in the hot sphere should fulfill EANM guidelines	Per scanner
Contrast media	15%	0%	Avoid pre-PET administration of IV contrast media. If contrast-enhanced CT is needed, IV contrast should be administered after low-dose CT for AC[d]	Per patient
Region of interest (ROI)	50%	0%	Statistical bias due to different methods of defining ROI for SUVs should be reduced by using the same algorithm for PET segmentation. Systematic bias could persist since no method assures to measure the "true" SUV of a lesion	
Uptake time	15%	8%	For clinical trials consistently use uptake time of 55' to 75' after injection	Per patient

Table 4.2 (continued)

Source of errors	Typical errors (routine)[a]	Expected errors (controlled environment)	Action to be carried out[b]	Performed
Motion and respiration artifacts	30%	–	Particular care should be devoted if quantitative measurements of lesions are carried out in the thoracic region. Use breathing control device if available	Per patient
Blood glucose level	15%	Unknown	Blood glucose level should be measured and reported. Guidelines should be used for managing hyperglycemia. Linear SUV correction is applied retrospectively	Per patient
Patient's weight	8%	2%	Patient's weight should be measured with 1 kg calibrated weight and reported	Per patient
Patient's height	–	–	Patient's height should be measured and reported for SUL calculation	Per patient

[a]Typical errors, such those encountered in routine clinical practice
[b]If proper actions are carried out, as listed in the last column, the errors could be reduced to the value indicated in column 3
[c]Acquisition and reconstruction parameters
[d]Attenuation correction

minimize SUV variability. The procedure for calibration of the PET scanner is depicted in Fig. 4.2. Although cumbersome, this approach proved effective in increasing the accuracy of tracer uptake measurements by 5–10% [6]. This is well below the range of 10–25% observed variations even in a controlled environment of a multicenter clinical trial [4]. Particular care should be taken to use the same activity calibrator to measure the activity used for calibrating the scanner. If more than one calibrator is used, they should all be cross-calibrated with a traceable radioactive source. PET sites not equipped with dose calibrators cannot get reliable SUV measures. Indeed, the activity injected in the patient must be always measured with the calibrator that is cross-calibrated with the PET/CT scanner used for imaging. If the activity is measured elsewhere, for example, at the radiopharmaceutical production site, this process is not necessary. Cross calibration in a multicenter framework generally permits to achieve a variability less than 10%, while 5% should be a requirement for using PET/CT in a quantitative way [7, 8]. An optimal inter-scanner variability of 3% has been reached when comparing two [8] PET/CT scanners requiring new cross-calibration strategies. Imaging parameters, such as scan duration per bed position, acquisition mode, ^{18}F-FDG dose, and reconstruction methods directly affect the image quality and quantitative results [3]. These parameters should be preset to fulfill the guidelines [1] for the recovery coefficient curve. The recovery coefficients are calculated as the ratio of measured and expected activity concentration in hot spheres of different radius in a phantom (Fig. 4.3). In addition to the above parameters, the actual administered activity and the accuracy of patient's weight and height influence the variability in SUV measurements. The injected activity is the difference between activity measured with the activity calibrator in the syringe and the syringe and administration lines residual. If the line is flushed with saline, the residual activity is usually lower than 1–3 MBq, and its measurement could be definitively omitted. Clock synchronization should be carried out on all the clocks of the department with respect to the scanner and the dose calibrator clocks to avoid bias in time and, consequently, SUV assessments.

Fig. 4.2 PET scanner calibration.
PET scanner electronics measure the
count rate of annihilation events.
PET scanner calibration is carried
out to associate an activity to this
count rate. This is done by injecting
a known activity, measured in an
activity calibrator, in a cylindrical
uniform phantom and scanning it
with PET

Prepare a syringe of a
beta+ emitter

Measure in a dose
calibrator

Inject in a phantom

Calculate the expected
activity concentration in
kBq/ml

Acquire the phantom on
PET/CT scanner and
measure activity counts

Associate counts/ml to
kBq/ml

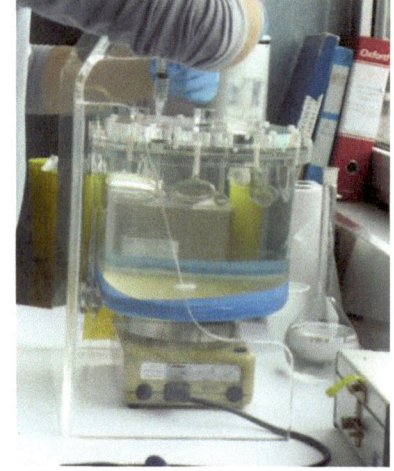

Data are given to reproduce the curves

x	Min	Max	opt	non opt
10	0.29	0.52	0.44	0.54
13	0.51	0.74	0.65	0.65
17	0.75	0.94	0.92	0.9
22	0.77	1.01	0.97	0.8
28	0.85	1.05	1	0.96
37	0.88	1.08	1	1

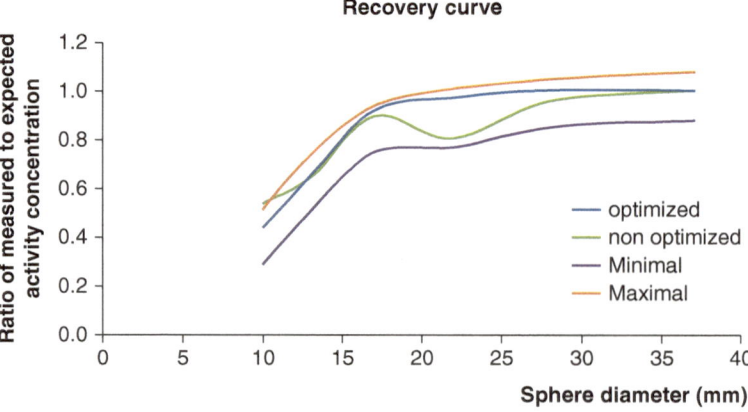

Fig. 4.3 Recovery coefficient.
An example of a recovery
coefficient curve is provided for
non-optimized (*left*) and
optimized (*right*) PET
parameters

Intravenously administered contrast media could alter SUV of a lesion if a diagnostic CT is performed as part of the PET/CT [3]. While specific recommendations could be found elsewhere [3], a general recommendation is to perform low-dose scan CT for attenuation correction before the PET scan and the full dose diagnostic CT after the PET scan. For the calculation of SULs, the patient's weight should be routinely entered in the PET dicom dataset with the calibration factors to avoid errors in SUV calculations (e.g., 5 kg difference in an 80 kg patient lead to a 5 % error in SUV).

Host Factors

Several patient-dependent factors from patient preparation to scan acquisition affect SUVs and must be verified on the single patient (Table 4.2). The biological factors include uptake time, plasma glucose levels, and patient motion or breathing artifacts. For most of these factors, clear recommendations [3] have been provided, as they directly affect SUVs and also image interpretation. In addition, SUV measurements are affected by tumor perfusion and hypoxia, inflammatory cell infiltrates in the tumor microenvironment, which cannot be controlled by extrinsic manipulations. The SUVs decrease in normal tissues with the increase of uptake time [9] with a linear decrease of SUV in all three compartments. The FDG uptake from the same lesion in images acquired at different time intervals after the radiotracer injection is influenced by the recirculating FDG. It is, hence, fundamental to use the same uptake time for all time points when sequentially imaging the same patient to maintain intra-patient consistency and to reduce the uptake time changes in longitudinal scans. As a general recommendation, a patient requiring quantitative PET measurements should be scheduled as the first patient of the day to minimize delays in acquisition times, which occur frequently later in the day. Moreover, in order to get comparable data in longitudinal studies, the PET scanner technicians should annotate the actual uptake time, to ensure reproducible results in the next scans. Elevated plasma glucose levels result

in decreased FDG uptake by the tumor, leading to erroneously low SUV values [1, 8]. Consequently, variable plasma glucose levels in longitudinal studies of the same patient will likely cause artificial SUV changes. A constant plasma glucose level in the range of 4–7 mmol/L in an individual patient across all longitudinal studies and tracks of the measured values are an achievable goal with a concerted team effort. There are several strategies for dealing with plasma glucose levels in SUV calculations, but further research is needed to understand whether intra-subject or inter-subject standardization is required. Patient's physical or breathing motion can also significantly influence SUV measurements [3]. To minimize this negative effect, the PET and CT fusion images should be visually analyzed to identify possible patient motion nearby a lesion. Patient breathing particularly influences the lesions in the thoracic area. Correction techniques are being introduced in PET/CT scanners using dynamic acquisition and breathing control devices; however, until then the data associated with motion should not be used for SUV measurements.

4.1.1.3 Metabolic Tumor Volume Measurements

Other proposed PET-derived functional metrics include metabolically active tumor volume (MTV) and total lesion glycolysis (TLG). The tumor volume concept has been developed in the late 1990s [10] but not evolved until recently because of the lack of necessary software developments. These volume-based PET parameters measure metabolic activity in an entire tumor mass designed to reflect tumor biology.

MTV

The MTV measure the total volume of the metabolically active tumor included within a VOI, both for a single lesion both for multiple lesions and expressed in cm^3 or ml. The rationale is the assumption of a metabolic activity higher than the surrounding healthy tissue to be able to accurately define the tumor volume. MTV is slightly affected by noise since it includes hundreds or thousands of voxels.

TLG

The TLG is the product of SUV_{mean} in the defined VOI and the MTV; the rationale is to combine tumor burden and its metabolic activity to obtain an index that is correlated to the tumor volume and the uptake within the entire volume. The routine application of these parameters is challenging because the quantification process requires complex calculations, is conducive to subjective definitions of VOIs, and is rather time consuming. There are several segmentation algorithm definitions, relying on manual (by an expert) or semiautomatic methods for tumor delineation (Table 4.3). With the recent development of software-assisted automated VOI assessments, volume-based metabolic quantitative parameters have become increasingly available. Although these metrics are potentially useful clinical

parameters for assessing treatment response and survival, they are not ready for clinical applications at the moment because they are yet to be standardized and validated [8–10]. The advantages and disadvantages of these methods are provided in Table 4.3.

4.1.1.4 Variability of PET-Derived Quantitative Metrics

The first prerequisite to reliably measure a PET-derived tumor volume is to assure a robust and reproducible method to accurately determine SUV-based parameters, overcoming the above-mentioned sources of error related to physical, technical, and biological factors [7]. In particular, all quantitative PET metrics are affected by user-defined factors including image acquisition settings, i.e., duration of acquisition, thickness of

Table 4.3 Pros and cons of the various categories of PET image segmentation techniques

Category	Characteristics	Limitations
Manual techniques	Visual interpretation and manual delineation of contours	Time consuming. Susceptibility to window level settings
	Very simple to use. Tools to transfer RT objects to treatment planning systems available from most vendors	Suffer from intra- and inter-observer variability. Consensus reading by nuclear medicine physician and radiation oncologist hardly practical in busy clinical departments
Thresholding techniques	Most frequently used due to their simple implementation and high efficiency	Hard decision making. Too sensitive to PVE, tumour heterogeneity and motion artifacts. Some methods focus on volume, others focus on intensity differences. Combination of both seems to provide best results [92]
Variational approaches	Subpixel accuracy, boundary continuity and relatively efficient. They are mathematically well developed and allow for incorporation of priors such as shape	Sensitive to image noise. As a PDE, stability and convergence could be subject to numerical fluctuations, especially if the parameters are not properly selected
Learning methods	Utilize pattern recognition power. Two main types: supervised (classification) and unsupervised (clustering)	Computational complexity especially in supervised methods, which require time-consuming training. Feature selection besides commonly used intensity is a flexibility but cab also be a challenge
Stochastic models	Exploit statistical differences between tumour uptake and surrounding tissues. Most natural to deal with the noisy nature of PET	Effect of initialization and convergence to local optimal solutions are concerns, especially when compromises are made to improve efficiency

Extracted by *Eur J Nucl Med Mol Imaging* (2010) 37:2165–2187, table 2, p. 2175 [32]

the slice, acquisition mode (2D vs. 3D), reconstruction algorithm, and the correction herein applied, i.e., attenuation, scattered and random coincidences, and dead time correction. To minimize SUV variability, it is necessary to cross-calibrate the PET scanners and ancillary instruments. Though cumbersome, this approach proved effective in increasing the accuracy of tracer uptake measurements, reducing inter-scanner variability of the measured activity to 5–10 % [7, 11–16], which is a major achievement, compared to 10–25 % variation observed even in a controlled environment of a multicenter clinical trial [17].

4.1.1.5 PET Test–Retest Reproducibility

Reported variability of SUV in patient test–retest studies differed from the desired range of ≤10 % [18–23]. The largest repeatability study of 62 patients with gastrointestinal malignancies reported an intra-subject coefficient of variation decrease in SUV measurements from 16 % to 11 % after applying a centralized quality control assessment and analysis [24, 25]. These studies showed that the variance of SUV is greater in clinical practice than in clinical trials even in a single site experience: the threshold criteria for a difference of a second scan in respect to baseline at 95 % confidence level were 49 % and 44 % for SUV_{max} and SUV_{mean}, respectively. A recent meta-analysis by De Langen et al. showed that SUV_{mean} had a slightly better repeatability than SUV_{max}, with a better reproducibility in larger lesions [26]. However, a recent study comparing SUV_{max}, SUV_{mean}, SUV_{peak}, and TGV found that different SUV definitions yielded 20 % variation in tumor response values for an individual tumor and variation of up to 90 % for a single SUV measurement [27]. Another study showed that mean percentage difference in SUV_{max} measurements in 100 patients with a known chest lesion obtained on subsequent scans was 0.9 ± 7.8 with a coefficient of variation of 4.3 % [28]. This variability was much lower than that reported in previous studies with a range of 2.5–8.2 % [7, 11, 29]. Besides SUV, Leijenaar et al. [30] demonstrated a high test–retest reproducibility of various radiomics features as well as a high (91 %)

interobserver variability. Based on the results of these studies, minimal protocol variation should be ensured when performing repeated scans on the same patient required to improve the reliability of SUV measurements.

4.1.2 Segmentation Methods for Volume Calculations

Different segmentation techniques for PET-derived volumes have been proposed with a varying complexity (Table 4.3). Hence, comparing the performance of different methods from published data is almost impossible given the variety of algorithms used and degree of operator manipulations [31, 32]. To date, there is no consensus on a reproducible, accurate, and practical method that should be preferred for tumor segmentation. The existing methodologies are described in the following paragraph.

Manual Technique The manual contouring by an experienced imaging expert is the first methods applied in this field and it is still widely used. However, this procedure is cumbersome, and time consuming, particularly in patients with disseminated disease. This method is technically least sophisticated but economically less demanding and expectedly leads to significant interobserver variability in the range of 5–137 % [33].

Thresholding Method The most widely used method to define a tumor volume is the thresholding method that requires identification of voxels exceeding a predefined threshold [34]. The thresholding can be performed using fixed or adaptive methodologies. In general, application of the proper threshold technique is a challenging task because of the limited resolution of PET images. Blurring due to partial volume effect [35] (Fig. 4.4) or motion artifacts and noise fluctuations due to limited photon counts can degrade segmentation accuracy.

Percentage threshold The earliest thresholding method was based on a percentage SUV, mainly using a cutoff of 40–50 % of the SUV_{max} [36].

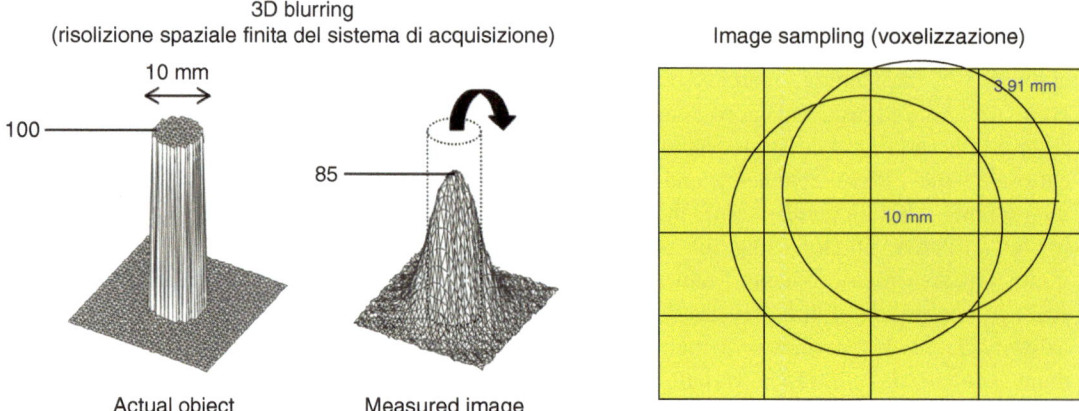

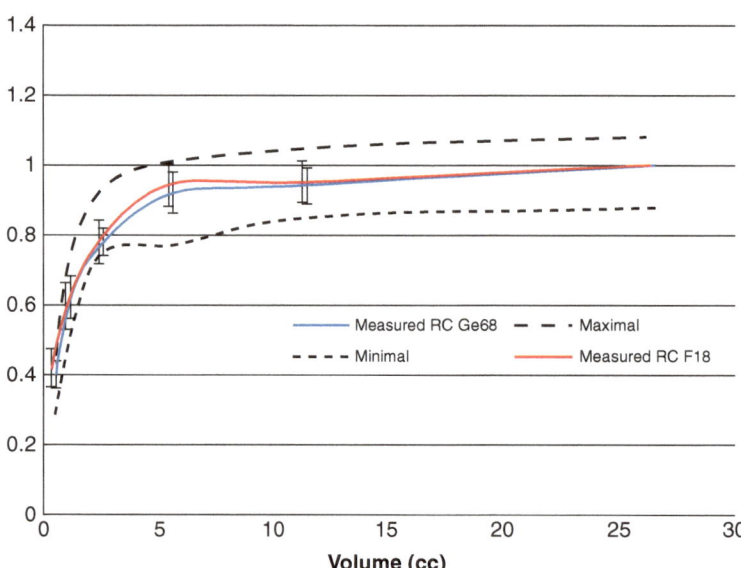

Fig. 4.4 Partial volume effect. Partial volume effect refers to both image blurring due to scanner finite spatial resolution (*left* in figure) and to voxel sampling (*right* in figure). It affects small lesions and is negatively affected by tumor heterogeneity. The SUV_{max} and SUV_{mean} measurements in a lesion volume of 2.5 ml (about 1 cm diameter) could be underestimated by up to 50 % (Fig. 4.2), and complete recovery of the actual SUV is done for lesions greater than 5 ml. Many strategies have been developed in the past to correct for partial volume effects but none of them reached a daily practice maturity [19]. Only recently, new algorithms have been applied directly to reconstruction algorithms in modern scanners. It should be emphasized that small tumor volumes do not necessarily imply small number of cells since the tumors become visible at about 10^5–10^6 malignant cells considering the resolution limits of the PET scanners

This method was simply based on phantom studies of static spheres. Subsequently, a value of 40 % was adopted by several groups for tumor delineation in radiotherapy planning of non-small cell lung cancer (NSCLC) [37], cervical cancer [38], and head and neck squamous cell carcinoma (HNSCC) [39]. The principal drawback of this method is that the optimal threshold is influenced by the size of the tumor volume; the surrounding background is not taken into account and is often "scanner specific" because of the strong dependence on the spatial resolution of the instrument. Based on the available data suggesting an insufficient tumor coverage using fixed thresholding methods, this method was no longer recommended, particularly for RT planning purposes [40].

Fixed threshold As an alternative method, an absolute SUV threshold can be used for tumor segmentation. However, tumor inhomogeneity and motion artifacts may hinder the application of this approach by failing to provide adequate tumor delineation in nearly half of the cases, in particular for lesions showing a low tumor-to-background ratio [41]. Moreover, fixed thresholding techniques take neither the background nor the tumor size into consideration [42] thus being inappropriate to define a tumor volume.

Adaptive threshold To address the background-dependent variability, some investigators suggested adapting the threshold to tumor-to-background (TBR) ratio [43, 44]. Subsequently, a more developed system based on an iterative technique was introduced to optimize the thresholding for the TBR approach [44–47]. The rationale is to change TBR threshold iteratively till when an optimal threshold is generated by the convergence algorithm. This is a reasonable and logic approach. However, the coexistence of several operator-dependent thresholding methods, based on different morphologic aspects of radiotracer concentration in tumors, justifies the search for an automatic threshold computing software.

Gradient technique This technique measures gradient differences between the lesion and the surrounding background with a good spatial accuracy and efficiency [48, 49]. Gradient methodology includes simple edge or ridge detectors [50] or watershed method [51]. More recently deformable active contour models have been applied to PET segmentation with the assumption that contours are characterized by sharp variations in the image intensity [52, 53]. Despite being intuitive, the gradient technique suffers considerably from image noise and often requires filtering of the images with a blurring effect [54].

More sophisticated techniques To overcome all the difficulties originating from thresholding and gradient techniques, several authors have explored more sophisticated approaches used in other science domains such as active deformable models, learning methods, and stochastic approaches [55] and those using a pattern recognition algorithm [56]. Learning methods based on classification require training of the method moving from data with known labels (known ground truth). However, this is a challenging task due to variability of PET tracer uptakes and biodistribution in tissues, which in turn depends on the biomarker concentration in the blood (e.g., glucose concentration for FDG) and other technical factors. In addition, PET images need to be properly drawn to identify the ground truth for training purposes (e.g., the structures contoured by a panel of experienced radiologists). Therefore, behind the ground truth, the application of these methods requires a number of other information with a thoroughly checked source. Stochastic models offer the advantage of incorporating the variable of the voxel's intensity directly into the model. However, these models are based on a proper predefined noise model, which has not been yet defined for PET and is strongly influenced by the parameters and type of the reconstruction algorithm. In general, the Gaussian assumption is used because it simplifies the computational burden and speeds up convergence.

Comparison between methods Reproducibility is a key issue associated with segmentation methods. Different methods give rise to variations in the calculated PET volumes in the range of 40–50 % [9, 31, 58, 59], and this variability can even reach 400 % [32]. The performance of tumor delineation methods, in turn, largely depends on variations in the TBR, image resolution, and image noise level. Evaluating the accuracy of the segmentation methods is rather difficult because it is virtually impossible to rely on a ground truth as comparator. Studies have been proposed using phantoms, morphological images (CT or MRI), and pathology specimens [57], but there is no consensus among scientists on the optimal method. Despite the heterogeneity of clinical behavior and aggressiveness of the malignant processes, there is preliminary evidence to suggest that MTV and TLG have independent prognostic value across different types of cancers, including lymphoma [60]. It is therefore important to pursue validation studies to establish the real value of these methodologies and also prove their reproducibility in large prospective data sets.

4.1.2.1 Applications in Radiation Oncology

Radiation therapy (RT) is one of the pillars of combined-modality treatment for the Hodgkin lymphoma. Successive technological progresses achieved over the past decade have revolutionized the definition of the target tumor volume and the boundaries of the radiation field. These new methods increased the effectiveness of this treatment modality which delivered much smaller doses to critical organs such as the lung, heart, and breast [61]. RT treatments can be classified as total lymphoid/nodal irradiation (TLI/TNI), extended field RT (EFRT), involved-field RT (IFRT), and involved node RT (INRT) (see Chapter 5). In the modern era of conformal radiotherapy, TNI and the EFRT are no longer in practice and supplanted by limited-field radiation therapy: IFRT, if the RT field encompasses all of the clinically involved nodal regions, and INRT, with an assumption to deliver the dose only to the initially involved nodes, rather than including the entire region of the involved nodal chain. Consequently, the current guidelines for combined chemotherapy and RT indicate that the delineation of the target volume should always be carried out on the affected regions [62, 63].

Field delineation in RT planning is one the most important applications of PET/CT imaging (see Chapter V). In recent years, a large number of studies and methodological research projects were performed to develop and validate automatic and semiautomatic algorithms for accurate and robust delineation of RT target volumes. So far only a few clinical trials have been conducted in which dose escalation was prescribed on an FDG avid area within the GTV [64–67].

Recent studies proved high observer variability in clinical target volume (CTV) delineation for HL [68–70], thus, highlighting the need for a robust and operator-independent methodology

for target definition. A considerable improvement in treatment volume definition on simulation CT has been obtained by integrating the information provided by the FDG-PET/CT, acquired before chemotherapy for diagnosis and staging purposes [67, 71–74]. In order to combine the FDG-PET/CT outcome with the CT-based CTV delineation, the common practice is the visual assessment. Briefly, the physician compares the two imaging modalities displayed on two different screens and confirms the matching on anatomical landmarks. However, this approach is time consuming and operator dependent. Some authors proposed methods based on rigid image coregistration and overlay (image fusion) highlighting favorable results if the FDG-PET/CT is acquired in the treatment position [73–75].

Dedicated PET/CT planning is already available in some centers, but care must be taken when fusing diagnostic and planning scans because of the need for a deformable registration, which is yet to become a standardized procedure. Nonetheless, there are practical obstacles in routine practice such as the scanning position of the patient (position of the arms and/or neck) and the use of different scanners. In addition, weight loss and lymph node shrinkage occurring between the two imaging stages represent particularly challenging issues for PET/CT matching based on rigid registration.

Similar to other cancers, PET/CT manual contouring is the standard technique in lymphoma [76]. To increase reproducibility, the use of a flat table for PET/CT imaging is advisable. Due to the relatively simple geometry of the lymphoma lymph nodal masses in axial CT and PET/CT sections, a PET segmentation algorithm has been rarely used instead of manual contouring for RT planning.

4.1.3 Conclusions

There is a large variability in computational complexity and level of user interaction required by the various image segmentation techniques. In the near future, the development of more sophisticated and robust tools for PET segmentation will probably help physicians to use these quantitative methods with higher precision and accuracy. However, it is imperative to adopt standardized acquisition, reconstruction, and analysis protocols for the clinical use of PET quantitative metrics.

4.2 Clinical Applications in Lymphoma

4.2.1 Why Should Quantitative Methodology Be Preferred Over Qualitative?

The widely utilized anatomic imaging parameters rely on tumor size change as a measure for treatment response. Nevertheless, functional imaging lends itself as a better surrogate metric for demonstrating a biological tumor response. Although visual assessment of FDG-PET/CT has been successfully integrated into clinical practice for therapy monitoring, high rate of false-positive results even in the hands of expert readers have raised concerns [77–81] for its usefulness, particularly, for interim PET-adapted therapeutic strategies. With the emphasis on the liver as a reference background adopted by D 5PS criteria [82], the inter-patient variability and intra-patient fluctuations of hepatic FDG uptake during therapy [83–85] have become a focus of concern. More importantly, the depth of tumor response categorization by visual criteria may lead to suboptimal differentiation between response categories by oversimplification. Furthermore, visual assessment is proven to be a reproducible and efficacious method for treatment response assessment in HL [159, 160] and FL [179] but its role is less substantiated with the currently available data in other lymphoma subsets [153]. Quantitative analysis allows for an objective assessment of treatment response, thereby minimizing interobserver variations and more suitable for a continuous measure of response which is also one of the most effective ways to reduce sample size [86]. In order to minimize potential treatment-associated morbidity, and unnecessary

interventions, the tumor metabolic response can be used as a practical early clinical end point to substitute survival end points, which may counteract the high cost and lengthy process attendant with the regulatory approval of the novel drugs. Functional imaging provides an earlier and faster readout for treatment response compared to morphologic imaging; consequently, it is preferable for early and accurate evaluation of the efficacy of novel treatments. With the recent insurgence of sophisticated software programs, tumor volumes can be determined with much less effort than otherwise. Thus, MTV as a measure of the viable tumor fraction or TLG, as a product of MTV and mean SUV within the volume, may better predict ultimate patient outcome than anatomical imaging either at baseline or early during therapy. MTV is and may better estimate tumor burden. Hence, there is a strong interest in the development of various quantitative metabolic PET metrics in an effort to decrease the rate of false-positive results, increase reproducibility, and maximize statistical power.

4.2.2 PET-Derived Quantitative Metrics in Clinical Practice

4.2.2.1 Standardized Uptake Values (SUV)

As alluded in the previous section, SUV_{max} has been investigated as a quantitative PET parameter to provide an objective measure for assessing tumor metabolic activity in tissues.

Baseline Tumor Characterization

The advent of genomic and proteomic technologies have been shifting traditional cancer management toward an individualized treatment strategy. However, these methods are impractical in a routine setting and do not allow for a complete characterization of the tumor because tumor tissues are spatially and temporally heterogeneous. Noninvasive assessment of tumor behavior with the use of imaging may provide a more comprehensive guidance for improving therapy decisions in cancer patients. Among all indications, differentiation between a malignant and benign etiology or a low-grade phenotype from that of a high grade using an objective imaging tool would be clinically desirable. In this regard, although limited and not validated, the existing published data showing correlation between the SUV_{max} and tumor histologic characteristics, surgical stage, and prognosis are summarized in the following section.

Diagnosis of different tumor phenotypes Considering the need for a more aggressive treatment for transformed low-grade lymphomas (LGL) compared to LGLs [87], early identification of transformation to an aggressive phenotype would be clinically consequential. There is sufficient evidence that FDG-PET/CT can detect transformation of chronic lymphocytic leukemia (CLL) to diffuse large B-cell lymphoma (DLBCL), the so-called Richter's transformation [88–91]. In a retrospective study by Bruzzi et al. ($n=37$), SUV_{max} of >5.0 was considered highly suggestive of Richter's transformation with an overall sensitivity and negative predictive value (NPV) of 91% and 97%, respectively [88]. Recently, Falchi et al. evaluated and reported that SUVmax ≥ 10, international prognostic score (IPS) ≥ 2, bulky disease, and age ≥ 65 were independently associated with shorter OS in CLL patients ($n=332$) [89]. $SUV_{max} \geq 10$ strongly correlated with overall survival (OS) (OS: 57 vs. 7 months). Corroborating these results, Michallet et al. identified a threshold of tumor SUV_{max} >10 as the most effective discriminating cutoff value which yielded a sensitivity and specificity of 91% and 95%, respectively, for identifying transformation by PET in CLL patients ($n=250$) [90].

The transformation to large B-cell aggressive lymphoma is also a critical event for patients with follicular lymphoma (FL), which warrants a more aggressive therapy approach than de novo FL. The value of FDG-PET/CT diagnosing transformation has been well established for guiding lymph node biopsy when transformation is suspected. Although there is lack of consistency for defining an exact SUV_{max} cutoff, a transformation is suggested at a SUV_{max} of 10–15 [91–96]. But it

should be emphasized that thresholds indicating transformation should be investigated in homogeneous patient cohorts because the cutoff value will be different for different subtypes of indolent lymphomas [94]. Because proliferation is a hallmark of transformation, 3'-deoxy-3'-[^{18}F]fluorothymidine (FLT), as a specific surrogate for proliferation [97], is hypothesized to be superior to FDG for early detection of progression to a more aggressive histology (see Chapter 1: the newer tracers). Nonetheless, there are conflicting reports and this premise has not yet been proven [95, 98]. In a comparative study ($n=26$) by Wondergem et al., the ability of FDG to discriminate between FL and transformed FL was superior to that of FLT with a SUV_{max} of 14.5 aiming at 100% sensitivity with a maximum specificity (82%) [95]. At the optimal sensitivity, the specificity of FLT was only 36% that would imply an unacceptably high proportion of patients requiring a biopsy to exclude transformation. The poor performance of FLT begs the question of its specificity for cell proliferation or Ki-67 expression. Therefore, the clinical impact of FLT remains to be determined in ongoing research studies.

The nodular lymphocyte predominant HL (NLPHL) is an uncommon subtype that invariably expresses CD20 with excellent OS, but unlike classical HL (cHL), late relapses may occur. In addition to staging and response assessment, determination of a disparate phenotype may be clinically relevant to because NLPHL has a propensity to be associated with concurrent or transformation to an aggressive B-cell non-Hodgkin lymphoma that would require long-term follow-up and image-guided rebiopsy. Hence, recognizing the imaging features of this entity is important. NLPHL is FDG avid, although SUVs are generally lower than those observed in cHL [99, 100]. A study by Hutchings et al. (n=60) found that the mean SUV_{max} was 8.0 vs. 11–15 for cHL, $p=0.002$ [99]. In a retrospective design ($n=12$), NLPHL patients were also found to have lower FDG SUV_{max} compared to those with T-cell/histiocyte-rich large B-cell lymphoma (THR-LBCL) (mean SUV_{max}, 6.9 vs. 16.6, $p=0.055$) [101].

Tumor heterogeneity The spatial and temporal tumor heterogeneity limits the accuracy of tissue-based molecular assays. However, algorithms of image characterizations may capture intratumor heterogeneity as a signature of gene expression patterns, particularly, with the use of quantitative methods [102, 103]. The heterogeneity of tumor morphology largely accounts for an idiosyncratic treatment response within a single or across different neoplastic disorders. Genetic and epigenetic differences between cancer cells within a tumor might explain why some tumor cells are resistant to therapy, while others are sensitive and can be eradicated after an effective treatment.

Radiomics is an emerging field and refers to the comprehensive evaluation of the entire tumor volume using quantitative image evaluation of tumor phenotypes [102, 104, 105]. Recently, the data published by Aerts et al. suggested that radiomics decoded a general prognostic phenotype existing in multiple cancer types by revealing associations with the underlying gene expression patterns [106]. In one series of mixed cancers including DLBCL, integrating image textural features with SUV measurements significantly improved the prediction accuracy of morphological changes (Spearman correlation coefficient=0.87, $p < 0.0002$) [107]. Some of the textural image features (such as entropy and maximum probability) were superior in predicting morphological changes of radiotracer uptake regions longitudinally, compared to SUVmax. In another pilot study, voxel distribution of FDG uptake demonstrated no significant differences in the heterogeneity indices between responders and nonresponders, while the heterogeneity of the intratumoral distribution of ^{111}In-ibritumomab tiuxetan was correlated with the tumor response in this cohort of 16 NHL patients [108]. In this study, pre-therapeutic FDG SUVmax was predictive of the tumor response to ^{90}Y-ibritumomab tiuxetan therapy on a lesion-by-lesion basis. This result is consistent with a previous report [109], while in another prior report, pre-therapeutic FDG SUVmax was not predictive of the tumor response to ^{90}Y-ibritumomab tiuxetan therapy [110]. This may be because of the small number of patients and different analysis methods. Nonetheless, in radionuclide therapy, the nonuniformity of the absorbed dose by the tumor may be a key issue for treatment success or failure. Pre-therapeutic FDG SUVmax in combination with heterogeneity of ^{111}In-ibritumomab tiuxetan might enhance the predictive values for tumor response and long-term outcome, which will be clarified in further studies. Radiomics may have a large clinical impact providing a wealth of extractable additional information that can be quantified for monitoring phenotypic changes during treatment. However, it is still in an early phase of development, and there are multiple technical issues that still need to be streamlined and validated to prove its clinical relevance.

Assessment of Bone Marrow Involvement (BMI)

Although it is widely recognized that a unilateral iliac crest BMB could underestimate lymphoma infiltration, bone marrow biopsy (BMB) has been the standard conventional method to evaluate bone marrow (BM) involvement in lymphomas (see Chapter 1: the need for bone marrow biopsy). However, BMB is associated with complications such as bleeding, anxiety, and pain [111, 112]. To overcome these disadvantages, the high sensitivity provided by whole body PET/CT imaging is exploited for effectively diagnosing BMI. According to the new Lugano guidelines, if a PET/CT is performed, a BMB is no longer required for the routine evaluation of patients with HL because of the low incidence of BMI [113, 114]. In DLBCL, if the scan is negative, a BMB is indicated to identify involvement by discordant histology if relevant for a clinical trial or patient management [113, 115, 116]. Several studies investigated whether visual and quantitative PET-based BM assessment can replace blind BMBs in various lymphoma subtypes.

Non-Hodgkin Lymphoma Adams et al. reported the inability of FDG-PET/CT to replace BMB in newly diagnosed DLBCL because PET-based BM assessments, including SUVs, were prognostically inferior to BMB ($n = 78$). Multivariate analysis showed that only BMB status was an independent predictive factor of PFS ($P=0.016$ and OS $P=0.004$) [117]. The design of this study, however, was not optimal because of retrospective analysis and the use of BMB as the only reference standard for the diagnosis of BMI, which only allowed for the calculation of patient-based sensitivity of FDG-PET/CT. The same group of investigators subsequently reported that head-to-head comparison with BMB, the diagnostic value of both visual and quantitative PET/CT for the detection of BMI, is low in a cohort of 40 DLBCL patients [118]. The SUV_{mean}, SUV_{max}, and SUV_{peak} of BMB-negative patients (1.4 ± 0.49, 2.2 ± 0.69, and 1.7 ± 0.59, respectively) considerably overlapped with those of BMB-positive patients (1.8 ± 0.53, 2.7 ± 0.71, and 2.2 ± 0.61, respectively).

Contrary to these results, in patients with FL, quantitative PET analysis was more beneficial in diagnosing BMI than visual assessment in a preliminary study of 22 patients. Optimal SUV_{max} cutoff of 2.1 yielded sensitivity and specificity combinations of approximately 87% [119]. In another study, of 41 patients with grade 1-3a FL and diffuse BM uptake, using a SUV_{mean} cutoff of ≥2 resulted in approximately 30% improved sensitivity at no cost to specificity. Moreover, using the ratio $SUV_{mean}/MBP \geq1$, the sensitivity of PET/CT to detect BM involvement improved to 83% [120]. As a limitation, this study was retrospective and included both staging and restaging patient groups which added heterogeneity to the data.

Hodgkin lymphoma Although the value of qualitative analysis and the rareness of BMI in HL have been addressed previously, several studies investigated the added value of a quantitative PET approach in the detection of BMI by HL. SUV_{max} evaluation did not have an incremental value to the visual evaluation in a retrospective study included 26 HL patients [121]. In another retrospective study of 106 HL patients, Salaun et al. reported that multivariate analysis revealed an independent correlation between sacral SUV_{max} and Ann Arbor stage ($p=0.005$). No BMI was found in patients who presented with SUV_{max} below 3.4 [122].

In summary, because the qualitative interpretation of PET may be marred by the physiologic accumulation of FDG within the BM, there is a need for an objective whole body technique to yield quantifiable results that may simulate BMB. At first glance, the distinction between these potentially overlapping conditions may be easy, considering that only focal FDG uptake is considered to represent BMI in HL [113, 114]. However, this distinction is challenging in NHL where BMI can present with both focal and diffuse patterns of FDG uptake [116, 117]. In this regard, development of a quantitative PET approach may be particularly relevant in patients with newly diagnosed NHL. However, a number of unsettled issues still exists, i.e., what extent of increase in BM uptake should be considered suggestive of BMI, if this increase could be quantifiable how should it be corrected by the actual BM volume that individually varies from one patient to another, how to factor in the differences in the BM volume in different parts of the body, and, finally, what would be the methods to minimize an overlap between reactive BM hyperplasia and diffuse BMI. With the wealth of available software programs, further work is underway to address these viable concerns to determine the actual role of a quantitative PET approach.

4.2.2.2 Quantitative PET-Derived Metrics Beyond SUVs

As discussed at length in the previous section, SUV can be biased by the count variability and tumor heterogeneity in a volume of interest because of the reliance on a single voxel measurement. Furthermore, besides the anatomic finding of high tumor burden in a disseminated disease, which is frequently recorded at baseline in lymphoma, a methodology able to assess and quantify the metabolic activity of a given tumor burden would be more clinically relevant. In an effort to reduce bias, increase reproducibility, and improve the predictive value of PET results, functional volume parameters, i.e., metabolic tumor volume (MTV) and tumor lesion glycolysis (TLG) have been under investigation [1, 8–10].

Prognostic Value of PET-Derived Quantitative Metrics at Baseline

If the baseline whole body disease volume is proven to be an independent prognostic factor, high-risk patients may be objectively identified for treatment intensification. However, there is paucity of clinical data for the establishment of a prognostic system that is based on pre-therapy quantitative PET metrics affecting clinical outcomes of lymphoma patients. The available literature in both HL and NHL is discussed in the following section and summarized in Table 4.4.

Hodgkin lymphoma Tumor bulk is a significant negative prognostic factor in early-stage HL [113, 123–125]. However, not only the exact definition of tumor bulk remains a controversial topic but also an objective method to measure whole body tumor burden is yet to be established for a patient-tailored management. Thus far, the practice has relied on the indirect measures of tumor burden, i.e., the extent of involved sites used by the Ann Arbor staging system, and integrated factors including number of disease sites, stage, and LDH used by the prognostic systems including the international prognostic score (IPS) to stratify risk categories [126–129]. In a prior study of HL patients treated on standard protocols, the mean tumor burden normalized to body surface area based on CT measurements was found to be largely superior to all prognostic models as a predictor of complete remission and survival [124, 125]. Given the coverage of the entire body, metabolic volume determination may be a better surrogate for response and survival by representing overall tumor functionality.

Several retrospective studies using various methodologies calculating the tumor volume showed that there may be a benefit to use PET quantitative metrics to predict survival [130–132]. In a study by Song et al. in 127 early-stage HL patients (20% bulky) treated with six cycles of ABVD, with or without involved-field radiotherapy (IFRT), the multivariate analysis showed that only older age, B symptoms, and high MTV status were independently associated with PFS

and OS (PFS, $p = 0.008$; OS, $p = 0.007$) [130]. In this study, a fixed threshold method of $\geq SUV_{max}$ 2.5 was used to determine the disease volume. In another single-center study, Kanoun et al. showed that pre-therapy MTV was predictive of patient outcomes in a cohort of 59 HL patients (92% stage II–IV, 60% IPS > 2), who were treated with an anthracycline-based therapy with or without IFRT [131]. The patients with a low MTV had a significantly better 4-year PFS than those with a high MTV (85% vs. 42%, p = 0.001, 88% vs. 45%, $p = 0.0015$, respectively). MTVs were measured with a semiautomatic method using a 41% SUVmax threshold. In multivariate analysis only baseline MTV ($p < 0.006$, RR 4.4) and ΔSUV_{max} at PET2 (71%, $p = 0.0005$, RR 6.3) remained independent predictors of PFS when tumor bulk (≥ 10 cm) did not reach statistical significance. In contrast to these findings, Tseng D. et al. reported that at a median follow-up of 50 months, baseline absolute PET metrics including SUV_{max}, SUV_{mean}, and MTV did not predict survival in 30 HL patients (stage IIB-IV 63%, 30% IPS > 2) treated with varying chemotherapy regimens with or without IFRT when IPS was associated with PFS ($p < 0.05$) and OS ($p < 0.01$) [132]. On the contrary, the ΔMTV ($p < 0.01$), ΔSUV_{max} ($p = 0.01$), and ΔSUV_{mean} ($p < 0.05$) at interim PET were associated with PFS and OS. This divergent result compared to others may be on the basis of a small patient cohort and the differences in methodologies, patient population, (stage, risk factors) and therapy protocol. However, all of the above reviewed studies had suboptimal designs marred by the retrospective design, which was inherently prone to biases because of non-standardized protocols and patient preparation (see previous section). Also the use of various segmentation methods and resultant MTV cutoffs that varied between 200 and 500 ml led to non-comparable and non-generalizable results. Moreover, a fixed threshold that was used by all of these studies is not considered optimal for volumetric assessment as discussed in the previous technical section.

In a retrospective analysis of prospectively acquired data in 89 cHL patients whose findings were reported previously by Hutchings et al.

Table 4.4 Published studies in lymphoma using metabolic tumor volume as a measure of outcome

	Patients	No. pts		Multicenter	Mono, multi or equalized scanners	Therapy	PET time	Segmentation method	Segmentation performed by	Cutoff
Kanoun et al. [131]	HL, excluding nodular lymphocyte predominant lymphoma	59	RE	No	MU (2 scanners)	4–6 cycles of an anthracycline-based chemo plus 20–36 Gy of IF-RT	Baseline, interim[2]	41 % SUV_{max} threshold, manual adjusted	2 blinded experts, consensus if discrepant	MTV 225 cm^3
Song et al. [130]	Early HL	127	RE	Yes	MU	6× ABVD plus 30 Gy of IF-RT plus 10 Gy on initial bulk	Baseline	Visual and fixed threshold of 2.5 SUV	Locally and reviewed centrally by an expert	MTV 198 cm^3
Tseng et al. [132]	Early and advanced HL,	30	RE	No	MO	Stanford V, ABVD, VAMP, or BEACOPP plus RT (20 Gy, 25.5 Gy, or 36 Gy)	Baseline, interim[2]	Region-growing algorithm[69]	–	NS
Hussien et al. [162]	Pediatric HL	54	PRO	Yes	EQ	GPOH-HD2002P, GPOH-HD2003, EuroNet-PHL-C1 plus IFRT	Baseline, interim2	D 5PS and fixed threshold of 2.5 SUV (body weight, body surface) and at a threshold of mean liver plus two standard deviations SUV (lean body mass)	Two blinded experts	
Esfahani et al. [137]	DLBCL	20	RE	No	MO	6× or 8× R-CHOP	Baseline, interim[2]	Threshold 1.5 liver SUV_{mean} plus 2.5 standard deviation of liver SUV. Contours were manually adjusted in case of tumor exceeding contrast-enhanced CT volumes	Two blinded experts	MTV=379, and 5.95 TLG=705 and 96.5 at baseline and at interim PET2, respectively

	No, pts								
Kim et al. [141]	DLBCL	140	RE	No	MO	6–8 cycles of R-CHOP plus 36 Gy of radiotherapy to bulky disease	Baseline	Visual and a percentage threshold at 25%, 50%, and 75% of SUVmax	Three experts	TLG (505)=415.5
Sasanelli et al. [140]	DLBCL	114	RE	Yes	MU	R-CHOP21, RCHOP14, and ASCT	Baseline	41% SUVmax threshold	One expert, subset of 50 by another	MTV 550 cm³ TLG-
Gallicchio et al. [145]	DLBCL	52	RE	No	MO	R-CHOP		Visual and percentage threshold of 42%	Three blinded experts in consensus for visual and subsets of 18 patients in double for segmentation	MTV 16.1 cm³ TLG 589.5
Adams et al. [146]	DLBCL	73	RE	No	MO, EQ with NEMA/IEC IQ	R-CHOP	Baseline	40% of the SUVmax	Single blinded expert	MTV 272.3 cm³ TLG 2955.4
Tateischi et al. [170]	Relapsed or refractory DLBCL	55	PRO	Yes	EQ [27] with NEMA/IEC IQ phantom	Bendamustine–rituximab	Baseline, interim2, and EoT	Visual with D 5PS and fixed threshold of 2.5 SUV	Two blinded experts, third if discrepant	Δ66–68% at interim 2 and Δ61–66% at EoT for MTV and TLG
Malek et al. [167]	DLBCL	140	PRO			R-CHOP or R-DA-EPOCH	Interim (2–4 cycles)	D 5PS, a 37% threshold of SUVmax and a gradient technique method	One expert	ΔSUVmax>72% and ΔMTV 52%
Ceriani et al. [151]	PMBCL	103	PRO	Yes	MU	R-CHOP and R-VACOB-P and IFRT	Baseline	25% threshold of SUVmax, manually corrected	One expert centrally	MTV =703 cm³, TLG 5814

No, pts number of patients, *MTV* metabolic tumor volume, *TLG* total lesion glycolysis, *D 5PS* Deauville 5-point score

[133], during a median follow-up was 52 months, no baseline clinical parameters correlated with PFS but both baseline and interim quantitative PET parameters correlated with PFS [134]. The MTV was the strongest predictor of PFS at baseline ($p = 0.002$) and D-5PS at PET1 ($p < 0.0001$) (unpublished data). However, these data were obtained in a mixture of early- and advanced-stage patients, with as much as 54 % of the original series of 126 patients having a limited-stage disease (IA-IIB (Fig. 4.5)). Further investigations should include a more homogeneous data for definitive conclusions on the role of quantitative PET in the determination of HL outcomes. In view of the existing promising data, there is a need for more prospective large datasets to definitively determine the complementary or independent role of quantitative FDG-PET metrics at baseline for predicting prognosis and guiding treatment decisions in cHL.

Diffuse large B-cell lymphoma For NHL, there are no universally accepted or validated criteria for defining "bulky" disease, although 6 cm was suggested as the best cutoff for FL [135] and 6–10 cm for DLBCL [136]. A more streamlined and objective tumor burden measure would be preferred to better guide management. The pretreatment FDG-PET metrics have been investigated as a potential predictor of survival in patients with DLBCL treated with rituximab, cyclophosphamide, doxorubicin, vincristine, and prednisolone (R-CHOP) [137–146]. In a retrospective study of 169 patients with stage II–III (74 % IPI ≤2) de novo DLBCL, prior to R-CHOP therapy (6–8 cycles), Song et al. found in a multivariate analysis that the whole body tumor burden was a more important prognostic parameter for PFS than Ann Arbor staging (HR = 5.3; OS, HR = 7.0, both $p < 0.001$) [138]. MTV was defined with a thresholding intensity based on SUV_{max} ≥2.5. With a median follow-up of 36 months, the 3-year estimates of PFS and OS were significantly higher in the low MTV than in the high group (PFS, 90 % vs. 56 %; OS, 93 % vs. 58.0 %, both $p < 0.001$). The same group of investigators found similar results in 165 early-stage (71 % IPI ≤2) primary gastrointestinal DLBCL patients

[147]. During a median follow-up of 37 months, MTV was a better predictor of survival than SUV_{max} as determined by the receiver operator curve (ROC) analysis (0.92 vs. 0.70). Multivariate analysis revealed that a high IPI score ($p = 0.001$) and high MTV ($p < 0.001$) were independent prognostic factors for both PFS and OS, while other known prognostic factors were not significant. In another study of 140 DLBCL patients who received R-CHOP therapy followed by RT to bulky disease, after a median follow-up of 28.5 months, the TLG at the threshold of 50 % ΔSUV_{max} was significantly associated with PFS and OS (HR = 4.4; $p = 0.008$ for PFS and HR = 3.1; 95 % CI = 1.0–9.6; $p = 0.049$ for OS) [141]. High IPI score and Ann Arbor stage of III/V did not significantly shorten PFS. Similarly, in a retrospective study of 114 DLBCL patients [140] enrolled in previously reported International Validation Study [148], Sasanelli et al., using a 41 % SUV_{max} threshold, found that MTV was the only independent predictor of OS ($p = 0.002$) and PFS ($p = 0,03$) compared with other pre-therapy indices including tumor bulk (≥10 cm), LDH, stage, and age-adjusted IPI. The 3-year estimates of PFS were 77 % in the low metabolic burden group and 60 % in the high metabolic tumor burden group ($p = 0.04$), and prediction of OS was even better (87 % vs. 60 %, $p = 0.0003$). TLG failed to predict PFS and was less predictive of OS than MTV, in contrast to prior results. This multicenter study, however, was flawed by the absence of a protocol harmonization and cross-calibration of scanners across participating canters, variability of therapy protocols, and also the lack of comparative analysis between volumetric results and SUVs. More lately, Kim et al. reported that the higher MTV inferred a significantly inferior EFS compared with the lower MTV group during a median follow-up of 28 months in 96 DLBCL patients who were treated with R-CHOP [142]. In this study, MTV was defined with a fixed threshold of 2.5. There was no difference in EFS between patients with stage II and III patients ($n = 53$), but the higher MTV group showed significantly inferior EFS in this group of patients compared with the lower MTV group. Likewise, Xie et al. demonstrated that according

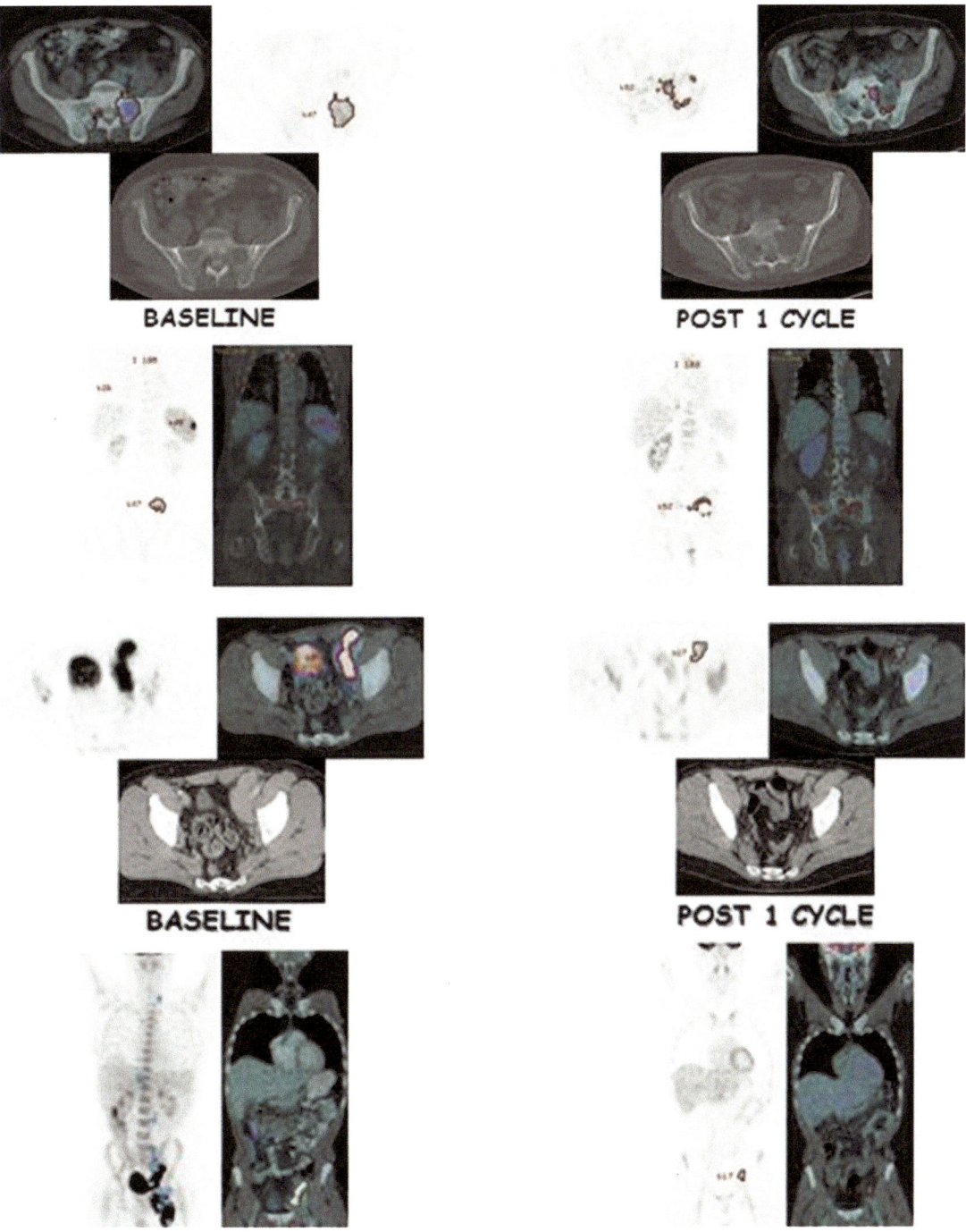

Fig. 4.5 Patient examples

to the cutoff determined from ROC analysis, lower MTV and TLG values prior to therapy were highly predictive of favorable PFS in DLBCL ($n = 60$) [144]. The multivariate analysis determined that the MTV and TLG values and number of enlarged lymph nodes predicted PFS independent of the National Comprehensive Cancer Network International Prognostic Index (NCCN-IPI) score and lactate dehydrogenase (LDH) level.

There are several studies whose results contradict with the previously reported studies [145, 146]. Gallicchio et al. suggested that the baseline SUV_{max} was a better predictor of EFS ($P = 0.0002$, HR 0.13) during a median 18-month follow-up than MTV and TLG in a study of 52 DLBCL patients with intermediate IPI scores, who were treated with R-CHOP [145]. Only the IPI score 3 was slightly but significantly associated with poor outcome. The metabolic volume was determined with a 42 % threshold. It is conceivable that patients with intermediate IPI score presenting high SUV_{max} would respond better since the magnitude of glycolytic activity rather than the amount of metabolically active burden appears to be the key determinant. Adams et al. retrospectively investigated the pretreatment PET/CT in 73 patients with newly diagnosed DLBCL who had undergone R-CHOP immunochemotherapy [146]. On univariate Cox regression analysis, only the NCCN-IPI was a significant predictor of PFS ($P = 0.024$), and only the NCCN-IPI and MTV were significant predictors of OS ($P = 0.039$ and $P = 0.043$, respectively). Therefore, the NCCN-IPI was suggested to remain the most important prognostic tool in this disease.

Combined results of a systematic review of seven retrospective studies involving 703 DLBCL patients [149] which included some of the above referenced studies [137, 138, 140, 141, 143, 146] suggested that SUV_{max} and MTV are significant prognostic factors for PFS (HR 1.61; $p = 0.038$ and 2.18; $p = 0.000$, respectively). Similarly, high MTV and TLG values unfavorably influenced the 3-year OS (OR, 5.40 and 2.19, respectively). For OS, only high MTV was a strong predictor of poor prognosis in DLBCL with HR 2.99

($p = 0.000$). Overall this meta-analysis found that the outcomes of the included studies were inconsistent. Although the principle treatment protocol in six trials was R-CHOP [137, 138, 140, 143, 146, 150], there were inhomogeneous treatments in one trial conducted by Sasanelli et al. [140] with 55 % of patients had received R-CHOP only, 45 % of patients had received R-ACVBP, and an additional 18 % of patients had undergone autologous stem cell transplantation. Additionally, the use of different risk scoring systems also impacted the homogeneity of the analysis. Five trials used the old IPI scoring system for risk stratification [137, 138, 141, 143, 150], one trial used the age-adjusted IPI scoring system [144], and the other used the recently proposed NCCN-IPI scoring system [146]. Except one study by Oh et al. [150], most patients of six trials had low-intermediate or high-intermediate risk according to IPI system. Thirdly, the varying inclusion and exclusion criteria might have led to the heterogeneity of the results. Moreover, each study varied widely in the optimal cutoff values for survival prediction, with the cutoff values ranging from 11 to 30 for ΔSUV_{max}, from 220 to 550 ml for MTV and from 415 to 2955 for TLG. The trials also differed in the Cox proportional hazard regression methods. Moreover, the small number of patients might have influenced the reliability of results. These are collectively the probable reasons leading to the high heterogeneity of the combined results. When the outcomes from other ongoing trials are published, a further meta-analysis will be needed.

In a prospective cohort of 103 primary mediastinal large B-cell lymphoma (PMBCL) patients enrolled in the International Extranodal Lymphoma Study Group (IELSG), Ceriani et al., reported that only TLG retained statistical significance for both PFS ($P < .001$) and OS ($P = .001$) in a multivariate analysis, who received combination chemo-immunotherapy [151]. The MTV was estimated using a threshold method based on 25 % of the SUV_{max}, which was lower than other proposed thresholds [132, 152]. The 5-year OS was 100 % for patients with low TLG vs. 80 % for those with high TLG ($p = .0001$), whereas PFS was 99 % vs. 64 %, respectively ($P < .0001$). Nonetheless, this was a retrospective evaluation in a group of 21 centers using various scanners. Additionally, despite a $p < 0.0001$, the HR for TLG was only 1.36 for increments of 10^3. Although considered preliminary, these results indicate that TLG at staging PET/CT could be a useful index in predicting outcomes in high-grade NHL including PMBCL treated with standard first-line chemotherapy regimens. Although it is premature to define the role of volumetric measurements in predicting outcomes, as a preliminary conclusion metabolic tumor volumes tend to be superior to ΔSUV_{max} in predictive values of survival, and a high MTV is significantly associated with reduced survival in DLBCL patients treated with R-CHOP. Because of the heterogeneity of the presently published data, these results should be interpreted with caution. This area of research will benefit from future large-scale prospective studies and further development in segmentation methodologies.

Predictive Value of PET-Derived Quantitative Metrics During or After Therapy

Taking a step forward from the traditional risk stratification systems, efforts have been concentrated on the interim PET results as a tool for guidance in early therapy modifications. However, the prognostic value of interim PET remains controversial in DLBCL patients with qualitative assessment variably correlated with outcome. The high false-positive rate associated with visual scoring systems, including the Deauville 5-point scale (D 5PS), has laid the grounds for quantitative PET initiatives when there is no existent optimal evaluation method for early assessment of response.

ΔSUV-based evaluation. Based on the results of multiple studies published by the Groupe d'Etude des Lymphomes de l'Adulte (GELA), it was suggested that the percentage reduction in SUV_{max} between baseline and interim PET (ΔSUV_{max}) improves both the interpretation accuracy and the interobserver reproducibility and better predicts patient outcome than visual analysis [153–155]. This group of investigators

demonstrated that a 66% reduction in SUV_{max} between baseline (PET0) and two cycles of chemotherapy (PET2) better predicted event-free survival (EFS) by reducing false-positive results of visual analysis. Other subsequent studies published corroborative results in DLBCL patients, treated with an anthracycline-based regimens plus rituximab [156, 157]. However, opposing results have also been reported by Pregno et al. in DLBCL patients treated with R-CHOP when the ΔSUV_{max} (both 66% cutoff and median) at PET2 to PET4 was rather weakly correlated with outcome ($p = 0.113$) [80]. Although it was in a homogeneous cohort, the limitation of this study included a small sample size, different time point analysis, and later than optimal time point preference (PET3 to PET4 vs. PET2). A similar quantitative approach was applied by Rossi C et al. to HL patients and showed that ΔSUV_{max} at PET2 was more accurate than the D 5PS in the prediction of outcome [158]. In this retrospective cohort of 59 consecutive HL patients who were treated with 4–8 cycles of anthracycline-based chemotherapy, PET2 $\Delta SUV_{max} > 71\%$ was considered a favorable response. Although visual PET2 positivity was related to a lower 4-year PFS (45% vs. 81%, $p < 0.002$), ΔSUV_{max} was more accurate for identifying patients with different 4-year PFS (82% vs. 30%; $p < 0.0001$). In a multivariate analysis using the IPI and $\Delta SUVmax$ as covariates, ΔSUV_{max} remained the unique independent predictor for PFS (RR, 8.1 and $p = 0.0001$). Quantitative interpretation of PET may lend itself as a more pragmatic tool to guide clinicians in lymphoma management but, the results of available data only pointed to the need for larger prospective trials and optimization and standardization of criteria for interim PET evaluation to assess the real prognostic value of interim PET results.

Tumor metabolic volume evaluation Although ΔSUV_{max} measurements partially improve on visual criteria and decrease the rate of false-positive results, a uniformly applicable ΔSUV_{max} cutoff has not been established to accurately predict clinical outcome. One can hypothesize that volumetric quantitative PET metrics have a better predictive value early during therapy beyond that of ΔSUV_{max} as well as traditional risk factors in lymphoma. The results are summarized under two topics, "HL" and "DLBCL," respectively, in the following section. In general, a judicious approach should be adopted when reporting these studies because of the fact that the majority of these studies were retrospective, and no detailed information was provided on the quality assurance of the investigated data as well as on scanner calibration, image reconstruction algorithms, and patient scanning protocols (see previous section). Another flaw in design of prior studies included the presence of mixed population of early- and advanced-stage disease. It has been long established that Ann Arbor staging is one of the most important pre-therapy prognostication system and an essential component of prognostic models such as IPI and IPS. Therefore, evaluation of the additional value of PET quantitative metrics in distinct categories of early- and advanced-stage patients is necessary to derive a clinically meaningful prognostic information.

Hodgkin lymphoma PET-derived quantitative metrics can improve the robustness of response assessment for therapy adaptation in HL patients. There are several studies designed to address this objective [131, 132, 134]. The results of the study by Kanoun et al. revealed that both baseline MTV and ΔSUV_{max} at PET2 were independent predictors of PFS in a mixed early- and advanced-stage HL population [131]. The combination of MTV and ΔSUV_{max} made it possible to identify three subsets of HL patients with different PFS outcomes ($p < 0.0001$). These included ΔSUV_{max} >71% and MTV $\leq$225 ml, ΔSUV_{max} $\leq$71% or MTV >225 ml, and ΔSUV_{max} $\leq$71% and MTV >225 ml. In these three groups, the 4-year PFS rates were 92%, 49%, and 20% ($p < 0.0001$), respectively. In another retrospective study by Tseng et al., 30 HL patients (53% stages III–IV and 67% had IPS$\geq$2) were treated with varying chemotherapy regimens [Stanford V (67%), ABVD (17%), VAMP (10%), or BEACOPP (7%)] with or without radiation therapy [132]. Interim-treatment scans were performed at a median of 55 days from the staging PET. At a median follow-up of 50 months, baseline absolute PET parameters did not predict survival while the ΔMTV ($p = 0.01$), ΔTLG ($p < 0.01$), and ΔSUV_{max} ($p = 0.02$) were associated with PFS. In this study, all calculated PET parameters were further associated with OS. IPS was also associated with PFS and OS ($p < 0.05$ and $p < 0.01$, respectively). These results suggest that the chemosensitivity of the tumor as measured by PET early during treatment is more predictive of clinical outcome than the initial tumor bulk which gives further credence to prior validation studies [159, 160]. However, on the basis of inclusion of relapsed patients and various chemotherapy regimens inclusive of intensive treatments, these data are not conducive to reproducible results with firm conclusions. The quantitative PET results were also investigated in pediatric HL patients [161–164]. Similar to adult population, response assessment after two cycles improved the specificity of response assessment by 30% using ΔSUV_{max} with a cutoff of 58% [163, 164]. Contrary to these results, however, multiple other studies did not confirm the high predictive power of PET status early during therapy [79–81]. In a recent study by Hussien et al. in 54 pediatric HL patients treated on treatment optimization protocols, all quantitative PET measures (SUV_{max}, SUV_{mean}, MTV, and TGV) fared significantly better than the qualitative response assessment using D 5PS at PET2 [162]. ΔSUV_{max} was the most powerful predictor of treatment outcome (area under the curve, 0.92; $p < 0.001$). The tumor volumes were determined with a fixed threshold of 2.5 SUV and at a threshold of mean liver plus two standard deviations SUV. In this study, technical parameters were better controlled than other studies, all PET scanners were cross-calibrated, and scan protocols followed EANM guidelines. However, sophisticated volumetric PET measures did not perform significantly better than the previously proposed ΔSUV_{max} in early response assessment [1, 3]. In summary, in the pediatric HL population, similar to the adult population, these results are preliminary and larger cohorts are needed to investigate this observation for a better definition of the role of PET/CT imaging. Recently, Hasenclever et al.

used a continuous scale by assigning D 5PS categories to certain quantitative PET cutoff values using the quotient of SUV_{peak} of the area with the most FDG avid residual uptake and the ΔSUV_{mean} of the liver in 898 pediatric HL patients after two chemotherapy cycles [165]. The borderlines for D 5PS 3, 4, and 5 at quantitative PET values corresponded to 0.95, 1.3, and 2.0, respectively, and quantitative PET of <1.3 excluded an unfavorable response with a high sensitivity. This method warrants a prospective validation study to be potentially used in clinical settings.

Diffuse large B-cell lymphoma Several retrospective studies investigated the value of quantitative PET-derived metrics in DLBCL, with the majority of data showing encouraging results [166, 167]. Park et al. investigated ΔSUV_{max}, TLG and Δ after 2 or 3 cycles in R-CHOP-treated DLBCL patients ($n=100$) including 57 patients with an IPI score of 1–3: the absolute values of baseline and interim SUVs calculated as the sum of values from 5 lesions (SUV_{sum}) and interim ΔSUV_{max} were significantly correlated with PFS [166]. While the ΔSUV_{max} and ΔTLG after 2 or 3 cycles were not associated with prognosis, the segmentation algorithm was based on mediastinal blood pool (MBP) threshold, which might have yielded larger MTVs than other thresholding methods would yield. The result of this study, although retrospective in design, highlights the potential of a quantitative approach to better delineate patient risk groups, particularly, in those with IPI scores of 1–3 which consists of the overlapping risk categories in which true low-risk patients should be better separated from the high-risk group to individualize therapies. These results could serve as a basis for future studies for the use of PET/CT in clinical practice, as an adjunct to IPI. Gradient-based methods appear to be more accurate compared with source-to-background ratio methods for segmenting FDG-PET images [43]. Malek et al. performed a retrospective study to correlate the ΔMTV and ΔSUV_{max} on interim PET with PFS after 2–4 cycles in 140 DLBCL patients using a gradient-based method rendered assessment of a greater tumor volume compared with the threshold-based method [167]. During a median follow-up of 37 months and with the use of R-CHOP and R-DA-EPOCH (rituximab-dose-adjusted etoposide, prednisone, Oncovin, cyclophosphamide, hydroxydaunorubicin) as the first-line therapy, D 5PS did not correlate with PFS ($P=0.37$). Compared with the threshold-based method, the gradient-based method resulted in a statistically significant greater MTV in pretreatment, as well as interim PET images. However, no significant difference was noted between the two methods. ΔMTV predicted PFS better than ΔSUV_{max} as the AUC for ΔMTV was significantly larger compared with that for ΔSUV_{max} ($AUC^{\Delta MTV}$: 0.713 and $AUC_{\Delta SUVmax}$: 0.873; P: 0.0324). Briefly, ΔMTV by either method after initial treatment was a better predictor of PFS compared with ΔSUV_{max}. Further analysis also revealed the underlying importance of ΔMTV on interim PET to predict PFS for patients who had also achieved a significant ΔSUV_{max}. MTV assessment (by either gradient- or threshold-based methods) may provide a more optimal methodology to accurately predict PFS as it incorporates the metabolic and volumetric information as a measure of tumor burden. Contrary to the aforementioned results, in a cohort of newly diagnosed 73 DLBCL patients, Adams et al. showed that the NCCN-IPI [168] was the most important prognostic tool for PFS ($p=0.024$) and OS ($p=0.039$) compared to PET-derived metrics including SUV_{max}, MTV, and TLG [146]. In this retrospective study, the authors used a threshold setting of 40 % of the SUV_{max} for volume delineation by a single expert. Median values of SUV_{max}, MTV, and TLG were used as cutoff values for group discrimination. Compared to prior studies, these significantly different results might have stemmed from methodological differences, different patient populations, shortcoming of the use of non-cross-calibrated scanners, and the overestimation of MTV and TLG through the use of a retrospective cutoff value in ROC analysis. In a pilot study of pediatric NHL patients ($n=16$), Furth et al. showed a limited predictive value for PET2 due to considerably high false-positive findings, especially in patients suffering from bulky disease [169]. With a mean follow-up of

60.2 months, the Kaplan–Meier survival analysis revealed no significant differences in 5-year PFS neither for conventional imaging modality (CIM) (76.9 % vs. 66.7 %; $p=0.67$) nor for visual PET (85.7 % vs. 66.7 %; $p=0.34$) nor for ΔSUV_{max}-based analysis (88.9 % vs. 57.1 %; $p=0.12$). In relapsed or refractory DLBCL, in a multicenter clinical trial of 55 patients treated with benda-mustine–rituximab, Tateischi et al. demonstrated that the ΔTLG can be used to quantify the response to treatment and can predict PFS after the last treatment cycle [170]. In this study, scanners were cross-calibrated using a NEMA/IEC image quality phantom. MTV was calculated with a fixed threshold $SUV_{max} > 2.5$. The percentage change in all PET parameters except for the area under the curve of the cumulative SUV-volume histogram was significantly greater in complete responders than in non-complete responders after two cycles and after the last cycle. The percentage change of the sum of total lesion glycolysis after the last cycle (relative risk, 5.24; $P=0.003$) was an independent predictor of PFS. An early PET scan after two cycles of treatment can effectively predict the outcome in patients with DLBCL treated with rituximab and anthracycline-based chemotherapy by using either a visual or quantitative approach. If its validity is proven in prospective studies, the interim ΔSUV_{max} approach may better serve clinicians to design a risk-adapted therapeutic strategy in DLBCL patients.

Radiation Therapy (RT) Planning

A limitation of FDG-PET in RT for HL is the variability in delineation of tumor volumes. Automatic or semiautomatic segmentation methods including thresholding based on a percent tumor ΔSUV_{max} may decrease variability in tumor delineations, but there is limited data in lymphoma using tumor volume segmentation methodologies. In a preliminary study using 15–40 % ΔSUV_{max} threshold segmentation method, on average, there was a 7.6-fold increase in PET volume between 15 % and 40 % ΔSUV_{max} x. There was a clinically significant decrease in dose to normal structures when the involved site radiation therapy (ISRT) plans were generated

using the 15 % ΔSUV_{max} × volumes compared with the 40 % ΔSUV_{max} [171]. If these results can be reproduced, a streamlined approach may be developed using segmentation methods for conformal therapies. Moreover, the increased functional volume could be an artifact when contrast-enhanced CT is used for attenuation correction. In this case, it is recommended that the delineation volume using the relative or adaptive method should be preferred when contrast media are used for PET/CT [172].

The use of FDG-based PET data for target volume delineation in ISRT and IFRT planning requires a mindful utilization of automatic segmentation methods in conformal field designs such as ISRT, in which variations in pre-chemotherapy GTVs may lead to clinically significant changes as a result of different SUV_{max} thresholds. Clinical judgment is still required for the delineation of target volumes, and no segmentation method can reliably discern between FDG uptake caused by neoplastic processes and by physiological or inflammatory processes. The most accurate method for target volume definition in HL remains the manual generation of the volumes by a skilled radiation oncologist with input from a nuclear medicine physician when needed. This field is in evolution and further robust data are required to determine a reliable segmentation methodology to optimize treatment volumes and dose to normal structures.

4.2.3 New Technology

Magnetic resonance imaging (MRI) using diffusion-weighted technique (DWI) has been suggested as a useful method in the assessment of lymphoma lesions, particularly those with multiple conglomerate lymph nodes. There is preliminary evidence that the glycolytic rate as measured by FDG-PET and changes in water compartmentalization and water diffusion as measured by the apparent diffusion coefficients on DWI (ADC) are independent biological phenomena in newly diagnosed DLBCL [173, 174]. In one series, however, there was no significant correlation between ΔSUV_{max} and ΔADC after initiation of the first cycle of chemotherapy in patients with HL or DLBCL. Thus, these data did not support the replacement of FDG-PET with DW-MRI for response evaluation in lymphoma patients [175]. ADC values were also found to discriminate between indolent and aggressive NHL, and this finding can be useful in assessing possible transformation from indolent to aggressive NHL [176]. There is also pilot data showing that the accuracy of DWI was significantly higher than that with PET/CT for mediastinal and hilar lymphadenopathy in differentiating between malignant and benign conditions [177]. In other cohorts, DW-MRI provided results comparable with or complementary to those of PET/CT for staging and early response assessment in DLBCL [178–180].

In summary, the literature is not mature to definitively prove or refute a diagnostic role for this modality compared to PET imaging in lymphoma patients. Further studies are warranted to assess the complementary roles of these different imaging biomarkers in the evaluation and follow-up of lymphoma.

Conclusions

The quantitative assessment with PET-derived volumes is still evolving and these preliminary findings suggest that it can be potentially useful in the prediction of clinical outcome and may improve on the predictive value of conventional risk-stratifying systems. However, currently, there is significant heterogeneity in the published data on the prognostic value of quantitative PET; thus, these results should be interpreted with caution because of their limited retrospective design, insufficient representation of risk and stage groups, differences in treatment strategies, as well as the varying methodologies used to measure MTVs. Currently, there is no consensus regarding the most optimal quantitative index to assess the metabolical activity disease burden using PET/CT imaging. Hence, the prognostic and predictive value of functional tumor volume remains to be further investigated with standardized, prospective, multicenter studies to validate as to what extent these parameters could improve individualized treatment approach in lymphoma.

References

1. Boellaard R, O'Doherty MJ, Weber WA, Mottaghy FM, Lonsdale MN, Stroobants SG, et al. FDG PET and PET/CT: EANM procedure guidelines for tumour PET imaging: version 1.0. Eur J Nucl Med Mol Imaging. 2010;37:181–200.
2. Makris NE, Huisman MC, Kinahan PE, Lammertsma AA, Boellaard R. Evaluation of strategies towards harmonization of FDG PET/CT studies in multicentre trials: comparison of scanner validation phantoms and data analysis procedures. Eur J Nucl Med Mol Imaging. 2013;40:1507–15.
3. Boellaard R, Delgado-Bolton R, Oyen WJ, et al. FDG PET/CT: EANM procedure guidelines for tumour imaging: version 2.0. Eur J Nucl Med Mol Imaging. 2015;42:328–54.
4. Wahl RL, Jacene H, Kasamon Y, Lodge MA. From RECIST to PERCIST: evolving considerations for PET response criteria in solid tumors. J Nucl Med. 2009;50 Suppl 1(5):122S–50.
5. Lodge MA, Chaudhry MA, Wahl RL. Noise considerations for PET quantification using maximum and peak standardized uptake value. J Nucl Med. 2012;53:1041–7.
6. Boellaard R, Krak NC, Hoekstra OS, Lammertsma AA. Effects of noise, image resolution, and ROI definition on the accuracy of standard uptake values: a simulation study. J Nucl Med. 2004;45:1519–27.
7. Boellaard R. Methodological aspects of multicenter studies with quantitative PET. Methods Mol Biol. 2011;727:335–49.
8. Hatt M, Cheze-Le Rest C, Aboagye EO, et al. Reproducibility of 18 F-FDG and 3′-deoxy-3′-18 F-fluorothymidine PET tumor volume measurements. J Nucl Med. 2010;51:1368–76.
9. Cheebsumon P, Yaqub M, van Velden FH, et al. Impact of [(18)F]FDG PET imaging parameters on automatic tumour delineation: need for improved tumour delineation methodology. Eur J Nucl Med Mol Imaging. 2011;38:2136–44.
10. Larson SM, Erdi Y, Akhurst T, et al. Tumor treatment response based on visual and quantitative changes in global tumor glycolysis using PET-FDG Imaging. The visual response score and the change in total lesion glycolysis. Clin Positron Imaging. 1999;2:159–71.
11. Geworski L, Knoop BO, de Wit M, et al. Multicenter comparison of calibration and cross calibration of PET scanners. J Nucl Med. 2002;43:635–9.
12. Boellaard R, Hristova I, Ettinger S, et al. EARL FDG-PET/CT accreditation program: feasibility, overview and results of first 55 successfully accredited sites. J Nucl Med. 2013;54 Suppl 2:2052.

13. Zijlstra JM, Boellaard R, Hoekstra OS. Interim positron emission tomography scan in multi-center studies: optimization of visual and quantitative assessments. Leuk Lymphoma. 2009;50:1748–9.

14. Scheuermann JS, Saffer JR, Karp JS, Levering AM, Siegel BA. Qualification of PET scanners for use in multicenter cancer clinical trials: the American College of Radiology Imaging Network experience. J Nucl Med. 2009;50:1187–93.

15. Christian P. Use of a precision fillable clinical simulator phantom for PET/CT scanner validation in multi-center clinical trials: the SNM Clinical Trials Network (CTN) Program. J Nucl Med. 2012;53(Suppl):437.

16. Sunderland JJ, Christian PE. Quantitative PET/CT Scanner performance characterization based upon the SNMMI Clinical Trial Network oncology clinical simulator phantom. J Nucl Med. 2015;56:145–52.

17. Erlandsson K, Buvat I, Pretorius PH, Thomas BA, Hutton BF. A review of partial volume correction techniques for emission tomography and their applications in neurology, cardiology and oncology. Phys Med Biol. 2012;57:R119–59.

18. Weber WA, Ziegler SI, Thödtmann R, Hanauske AR, Schwaiger M. Reproducibility of metabolic measurements in malignant tumors using FDG PET. J Nucl Med. 1999;40:1771–7.

19. Krak NC, Boellaard R, Hoekstra OS, Twisk JWR, Hoekstra CJ, Lammertsma AA. Effects of ROI definition and reconstruction method on quantitative outcome and applicability in a response monitoring trial. Eur J Nucl Med Mol Imaging. 2005;32:294–301.

20. Minn H, Zasadny K, Quint L, Wahl R. Lung cancer: reproducibility of quantitative measurements for evaluating 2-[F-18]-fluoro-2-deoxy-D-glucose uptake at PET. Radiology. 1995;196:167–73.

21. Nakamoto Y, Zasadny KR, Minn H, Wahl RL. Reproducibility of common semi-quantitative parameters for evaluating lung cancer glucose metabolism with positron emission tomography using 2-deoxy-2-[18 F]fluoro-D-glucose. Mol Imaging Biol. 2002;4:171–8.

22. Nahmias C, Wahl LM. Reproducibility of standardized uptake value measurements determined by 18 F-FDG PET in malignant tumors. J Nucl Med. 2008;49:1804–8.

23. Takahashi Y, Oriuchi N, Otake H, Endo K, Murase K. Variability of lesion detectability and standardized uptake value according to the acquisition procedure and reconstruction among five PET scanners. Ann Nucl Med. 2008;22:543–8.

24. Velasquez LM, Boellaard R, Kollia G, et al. Repeatability of 18F-FDG PET in a multicenter phase I study of patients with advanced gastrointestinal malignancies. J Nucl Med. 2009;50(10):1646–54.

25. Kumar V, Nath K, Berman CG, et al. Variance of SUVs for FDG-PET/CT is greater in clinical practice than under ideal study settings. Clin Nucl Med. 2013;38(3):175–82.

26. De Langen AJ, Vincent A, Velasquez LM, et al. Repeatability of 18 F-FDG uptake measurements in tumors: a metaanalysis. J Nucl Med. 2012;53(5):701–8.

27. Vanderhoek M, Perlman SB, Jeraj R. Impact of different standardized uptake value measures on PET-based quantification of treatment response. J Nucl Med. 2013;54:1188–94.

28. Lindholm H, Brolin F, Jonsson C, Jacobsson H. The relation between the blood glucose level and the FDG uptake of tissues at normal PET examinations. EJNMMI Res. 2013;3(1):50. doi:10.1186/2191-219X-3-50.

29. Young H, Baum R, Cremerius U, et al. Measurement of clinical and subclinical tumour response using [18 F]-fluorodeoxyglucose and positron emission tomography: review and 1999 EORTC recommendations. Eur J Cancer. 1999;35(13):1773–82.

30. Leijenaar RTH, Carvalho S, Velasquez ER, et al. Stability of FDG-PET Radiomics features: an integrated analysis of test-retest and inter-observer variability. Acta Oncol. 2013;52:1391–7.

31. Tylski P, Stute S, Grotus N, et al. Comparative assessment of methods for estimating tumor volume and standardized uptake value in (18)F-FDG PET. J Nucl Med. 2010;51:268–76.

32. Zaidi H, El Naqa I. PET-guided delineation of radiation therapy treatment volumes: a survey of image segmentation techniques. Eur J Nucl Med Mol Imaging. 2010;37:2165–87.

33. Riegel AC, Berson AM, Destian S, Ng T, Tena LB, Mitnick RJ, Wong PS. Variability of gross tumor volume delineation in head-and-neck cancer using CT and PET/CT fusion. Int J Radiat Oncol Biol Phys. 2006;65(3):726–32.

34. Otsu N. A thresholding selection method from gray-level histograms. IEEE Trans Syst Man Cybern. 1979;9:62–6.

35. Soret M, Bacharach SL, Buvat I. Partial-volume effect in PET tumor imaging. J Nucl Med. 2007;48:932–45.

36. Erdi YE, Mawlawi O, Larson SM, Imbriaco M, Yeung H, Finn R, et al. Segmentation of lung lesion volume by adaptive positron emission tomography image thresholding. Cancer. 1997;80:2505–9.

37. Bradley J, Thorstad WL, Mutic S, Miller TR, Dehdashti F, Siegel BA, et al. Impact of FDG-PET on radiation therapy volume delineation in non-small-cell lung cancer. Int J Radiat Oncol Biol Phys. 2004;59:78–86.

38. Miller TR, Grigsby PW. Measurement of tumor volume by PET to evaluate prognosis in patients with advanced cervical cancer treated by radiation therapy. Int J Radiat Oncol Biol Phys. 2002;53:353–9.

39. Scarfone C, Lavely WC, Cmelak AJ, Delbeke D, Martin WH, Billheimer D, et al. Prospective feasibility trial of radiotherapy target definition for head and neck cancer using 3-dimensional PET and CT imaging. J Nucl Med. 2004;45:543–52.

40. Nestle U, Weber W, Hentschel M, Grosu AL. Biological imaging in radiation therapy: role of

positron emission tomography. Phys Med Biol. 2009;54(1):R1–25.

41. Brambilla M, Matheoud R, Secco C, Loi G, Krengli M, Inglese E. Threshold segmentation for PET target volume delineation in radiation treatment planning: the role of target-to-background ratio and target size. Med Phys. 2008;35:1207–13.

42. Black QC, Grills IS, Kestin LL, Wong CY, Wong JW, Martinez AA, et al. Defining a radiotherapy target with positron emission tomography. Int J Radiat Oncol Biol Phys. 2004;60:1272–82.

43. Daisne JF, Sibomana M, Bol A, Doumont T, Lonneux M, Grégoire V. Tri-dimensional automatic segmentation of PET volumes based on measured source-to-background ratios: influence of reconstruction algorithms. Radiother Oncol. 2003;69:247–50.

44. Jentzen W, Freudenberg L, Eising EG, Heinze M, Brandau W, Bockisch A. Segmentation of PET volumes by iterative image thresholding. J Nucl Med. 2007;48:108–14.

45. van Dalen JA. A novel iterative method for lesion delineation and volumetric quantification with fdg pet. Nucl Med Commun. 2007;28:485–93.

46. Nehmeh SA, El-Zeftawy H, Greco C, Schwartz J, Erdi YE, Kirov A, et al. An iterative technique to segment PET lesions using a Monte Carlo based mathematical model. Med Phys. 2009;36:4803–9.

47. Marr D, Hildreth E. Theory of edge detection. Proc R Soc Lond B Biol Sci. 1980;207:187–217.

48. Huertas A, Medioni G. Detection of intensity changes with subpixel accuracy using Laplacian-Gaussian masks. IEEE Trans Pattern Anal Mach Intell. 1986;8:651–64.

49. Drever LA, Roa W, McEwan A, Robinson D. Comparison of three image segmentation techniques for target volume delineation in positron emission tomography. J Appl Clin Med Phys. 2007;8:93–109.

50. Geets X, Lee J, Bol A, Lonneux M, Grégoire V. A gradient-based method for segmenting FDG-PET images: methodology and validation. Eur J Nucl Med Mol Imaging. 2007;34:1427–38.

51. Hsu C-Y, Liu C-Y, Chen C-M. Automatic segmentation of liver PET images. Comput Med Imaging Graph. 2008;32:601–10.

52. Li H, Thorstad WL, Biehl KJ, Laforest R, Su Y, Shoghi KI, et al. A novel PET tumor delineation method based on adaptive region-growing and dual-front active contours. Med Phys. 2008;35:3711–21. Erratum pp 5958.

53. Long DT, King MA, Sheehan J. Comparative evaluation of image segmentation methods for volume quantitation in SPECT. Med Phys. 1992;19:483–9.

54. Aristophanous M, Penney BC, Martel MK, Pelizzari CA. A 53. Gaussian mixture model for definition of lung tumor volumes in positron emission tomography. Med Phys. 2007;34:4223–35.

55. Belhassen S, Zaidi H. A novel fuzzy C-means algorithm for unsupervised heterogeneous tumor quantification in PET. Med Phys. 2010;37:1309–24.

56. Chiti A, Kirienko M, Grégoire V. Clinical use of PET-CT data for radiotherapy planning: what are we looking for? Radiother Oncol. 2010;96:277–9.

57. Kirov AS, Fanchon LM. Pathology-validated PET image data sets and their role in PET segmentation. Clin Transl Imaging. 2014;2(3):253–67. doi:10.1007/s40336-014-0068-9.

58. Nestle U, Kremp S, Schaefer-Schuler A, Sebastian-Welsch C, Hellwig D, Rübe C, et al. Comparison of different methods for delineation of 18 F-FDG PET-positive tissue for target volume definition in radiotherapy of patients with non-small cell lung cancer. J Nucl Med. 2005;46:1342–8.

59. Shepherd T, Teras M, Beichel RR, et al. Comparative study with new accuracy metrics for target volume contouring in PET image guided radiation therapy. IEEE Trans Med Imaging. 2012;31:2006–24.

60. Gallamini A, Zwarthoed C, Borra A. Positron Emission Tomography (PET) in Oncology. Cancers (Basel). 2014;6(4):1821–89.

61. Zaffino P, Ciardo D, Piperno G, et al. Radiotherapy of Hodgkin and non-Hodgkin lymphoma. A non-rigid image-based registration method for automatic localization of prechemotherapy gross tumor volume. Technol Cancer Res Treat. 2015. pii: 1533034615582290.

62. Specht L, Yahalom J, Illidge T, et al. Modern radiation therapy for Hodgkin lymphoma: field and dose guidelines from the international lymphoma radiation oncology group. Int J Radiat Oncol Biol Phys. 2014;89:854–62.

63. Illidge T, Specht L, Yahalom J, et al. Modern Radiation Therapy for Nodal Non-Hodgkin Lymphoma Target Definition and Dose Guidelines from the International Lymphoma Radiation Oncology Group, from the International Lymphoma Radiation Oncology Group. Int J Radiat Oncol Biol Phys. 2014;89:49–58.

64. van Elmpt W, De Ruysscher D, van der Salm A, Lakeman A, van der Stoep J, Emans D, et al. The PET-boost randomised phase II dose-escalation trial in non-small cell lung cancer. Radiother Oncol. 2012;104:67–71.

65. Heukelom J, Hamming O, Bartelink H, Hoebers F, Giralt J, Herlestam T, et al. Adaptive and innovative radiation treatment for improving cancer treatment out- come (ARTFORCE); a randomized controlled phase II trial for individualized treatment of head and neck cancer. BMC Cancer. 2013;13:84. doi:10.1186/1471-2407-13-84.

66. Madani I, Duprez F, Boterberg T, Van de Wiele C, Bonte K, Deron P, et al. Maximum tolerated dose in a phase I trial on adaptive dose painting by numbers for head and neck cancer. Radiother Oncol. 2011;101:351–5.

67. Girinsky T, van der Maazen R, Specht L, et al. Involved-node radiotherapy (INRT) in patients with early Hodgkin lymphoma: concepts and guidelines. Radiother Oncol. 2006;79:270–7.

68. Genovesi D, Cèfaro GA, Vinciguerra A, et al. Interobserver variability of clinical target volume delineation in supra-diaphragmatic Hodgkin's disease. A multi-institutional experience. Strahlenther Onkol. 2011;187:357–66.

69. Lütgendorf-Caucig C, Fotina I, Gallop-Evans E, et al. Multicenter evaluation of different target volume delineation concepts in pediatric Hodgkin's lymphoma. A case study. Strahlenther Onkol. 2012;188:1025–30.

70. Shikama N, Oguchi M, Isobe K, et al. Quality assurance of radiotherapy in a clinical trial for lymphoma: individual case review. Anticancer Res. 2007;27:2621–5.

71. Yahalom J. Transformation in the use of radiation therapy of Hodgkin lymphoma: new concepts and indications lead to modern field design and are assisted by PET imaging and intensity modulated radiation therapy (IMRT). Eur J Haematol Suppl. 2005;75(s66):90–7.

72. Hutchings M, Loft A, Hansen M, et al. Clinical impact of FDGPET/CT in the planning of radiotherapy for early-stage Hodgkin lymphoma. Eur J Haematol. 2007;78:206–12.

73. Terezakis SA, Hunt MA, Kowalski A, et al. [^{18}F] FDG-positron emission tomography coregistration with computed tomography scans for radiation treatment planning of lymphoma and hematologic malignancies. Int J Radiat Oncol Biol Phys. 2011;81:615–22.

74. Eich HT, Müller RP, Engenhart-Cabillic R, et al. Involved-node radiotherapy in early-stage Hodgkin's lymphoma. Definition and guidelines of the German Hodgkin Study Group (GHSG). Strahlenther Onkol. 2008;184:406–10.

75. Robertson VL, Anderson CS, Keller FG, et al. Role of FDG-PET in the definition of involved-field radiation therapy and management for pediatric Hodgkin's lymphoma. Int J Radiat Oncol Biol Phys. 2011;80:324–32.

76. Konert T, Vogel W, MacManus MP, et al. PET/CT imaging for target volume delineation in curative intent radiotherapy of non-small cell lung cancer: IAEA consensus report 2014. Radiother Oncol. 2015;116:27–34.

77. Gallivanone F, Canevari C, Gianolli L, et al. A partial volume effect correction tailored for 18 F-FDG-PET oncological studies. Biomed Res Int. 2013;780458.

78. Hatt M, Le Pogam A, Visvikis D, et al. Impact of partial-volume effect correction on the predictive and prognostic value of baseline 18 F-FDG PET images in esophageal cancer. J Nucl Med. 2012;53(1):12–20.

79. Moskowitz CH, Schöder H, Teruya-Feldstein J. Risk-adapted dose-dense immunochemotherapy determined by interim FDG-PET in Advanced-stage diffuse large B-Cell lymphoma. J Clin Oncol. 2010;28:1896–903.

80. Pregno P, Chiappella A, Bellò M. Interim 18-FDG-PET/CT failed to predict the outcome in diffuse large B-cell lymphoma patients treated at the diagnosis with rituximab-CHOP. Blood. 2012;119:2066–73.

81. Cashen AF, Dehdashti F, Luo J, et al. 18 F-FDG PET/CT for early response assessment in diffuse large B-cell lymphoma: poor predictive value of international harmonization project interpretation. J Nucl Med. 2011;52:386–92.

82. Barrington SF, Mikhaeel NG, Kostakoglu L, et al. Role of imaging in the staging and response assessment of lymphoma: consensus of the International Conference on Malignant Lymphomas Imaging Working Group. J Clin Oncol. 2014;32:3048–58.

83. Ceriani L, Suriano S, Ruberto T, et al. 18 F-FDG uptake changes in liver and mediastinum during chemotherapy in patients with diffuse large B-cell lymphoma. Clin Nucl Med. 2012;37:949–52.

84. Groheux D, Delord M, Rubello D, et al. Variation of liver SUV on (18)FDG-PET/CT studies in women with breast cancer. Clin Nucl Med. 2013;38:422–5.

85. Rubello D, Gordien P, Morliere C, Guyot M, Bordenave L, Colletti PM, Hindié E. Variability of hepatic 18 F-FDG uptake at interim PET in patients with Hodgkin lymphoma. Clin Nucl Med. 2015;40:e405–10.

86. Gagne J. Innovative research methods for studying treatments for rare diseases: methodological review. BMJ. 2014;349:g6802.

87. Tsimberidou AM, Keating MJ. Richter syndrome: biology, incidence, and therapeutic strategies. Cancer. 2005;103:216–28.

88. Bruzzi JF, Macapinlac H, Tsimberidou AM, et al. Detection of Richter's transformation of chronic lymphocytic leukemia by PET/CT. J Nucl Med. 2006;47:1267–73.

89. Falchi L, Keating MJ, Marom EM, et al. Correlation between FDG/PET, histology, characteristics, and survival in 332 patients with chronic lymphoid leukemia. Blood. 2014;123(18):2783–90.

90. Michallet AS, Sesques P, Rabe KG, et al. An 18 F-FDG-PET maximum standardized uptake value >10 represents a novel valid marker for discerning Richter's Syndrome. Leuk Lymphoma. 2015;24:1–10.

91. Conte MJ, Bowen DA, Wiseman GA, et al. Use of positron emission tomographycomputed tomography in the management of patients with chronic lymphocytic leukemia/small lymphocytic lymphoma. Leuk Lymphoma. 2014;55(9):2079–84.

92. Schöder H, Noy A, Gönen M, et al. Intensity of 18fluorodeoxyglucose uptake in positron emission tomography distinguishes between indolent and aggressive non-Hodgkin's lymphoma. J Clin Oncol. 2005;23:4643–51.

93. Bodet-Milin C, Kraeber-Bodéré F, Moreau P, Campion L, Dupas B, Le Gouill S. Investigation of FDG-PET/CT imaging to guide biopsies in the detection of histological transformation of indolent lymphoma. Haematologica. 2008;93:471–2.

94. Noy A, Schöder H, Gönen M, et al. The majority of transformed lymphomas have high standardized uptake values on positron emission tomography scanning similar to diffuse large B-cell lymphoma. Ann Oncol. 2009;20:508–12.

95. Wondergem MJ, Rizvi SN, Jauw Y, et al. 18F-FDG or 3′-deoxy-3′-18F-fluorothymidine to detect transformation of follicular lymphoma. J Nucl Med. 2015;56(2):216–21.

96. Novelli S, Briones J, Flotats A, Sierra J. PET/CT assessment of follicular lymphoma and high grade B cell lymphoma – good correlation with clinical and histological features at diagnosis. Adv Clin Exp Med. 2015;24:325–30.

97. Shields AF, Grierson JR, Dohmen BM, et al. Imaging proliferation in vivo with [F-18]FLT and positron emission tomography. Nat Med. 1998;4:1334–6.

98. Buck AK, Bommer M, Stilgenbauer S, et al. Molecular imaging of proliferation in malignant lymphoma. Cancer Res. 2006;66:11055–61.

99. Hutchings M, Loft A, Hansen M, Ralfkiaer E, Specht L. Different histopathological subtypes of Hodgkin lymphoma show significantly different levels of FDG uptake. Hematol Oncol. 2006;24(3):146–50.

100. Ansquer C, Hervouët T, Devillers A, et al. 18-F FDG-PET in the staging of lymphocyte-predominant Hodgkin's disease. Haematologica. 2008;93:128–31.

101. Barber NA, Loberiza Jr FR, Perry AM, et al. Does functional imaging distinguish nodular lymphocyte-predominant Hodgkin Lymphoma from T-cell/histiocyte-rich large B-cell lymphoma? Clin Lymphoma Myeloma Leuk. 2013;13:392–7.

102. Lambin P, Rios-Velazquez E, et al. Radiomics: extracting more information from medical images using advanced feature analysis. Eur J Cancer. 2012;48:441–6.

103. Chicklore S, Goh V, Siddique M, et al. Quantifying tumour heterogeneity in 18 F-FDG PET/CT imaging by texture analysis. Eur J Nucl Med Mol Imaging. 2013;40:133–40.

104. Kumar V, Gu Y, Basu S, et al. Radiomics: the process and the challenges. Magn Reson Imaging. 2012;30:1234–48.

105. Tixier F, et al. Intratumor heterogeneity characterized by textural features on baseline 18 F-FDG PET images predicts response to concomitant radiochemotherapy in esophageal cancer. J Nucl Med. 2011;52:369–78.

106. Aerts HJ, Velazquez ER, Leijenaar RT, et al. Decoding tumour phenotype by noninvasive imaging using a quantitative radiomics approach. Nat Commun. 2014;5:4006. doi:10.1038/ncomms5006.

107. Bagci U, Yao J, Miller-Jaster K, Chen X, Mollura DJ. Predicting future morphological changes of lesions from radiotracer uptake in 18 F-FDG-PET images. PLoS One. 2013;8, e57105.

108. Hanaoka K, Hosono M, Tatsumi Y, et al. Heterogeneity of intratumoral (111)In-ibritumomab tiuxetan and (18)F-FDG distribution in association with therapeutic response in radioimmunotherapy for B-cell non-Hodgkin's lymphoma. EJNMMI Res. 2015;5:10.

109. Lopci E, Santi I, Tani M, Maffione AM, Montini G, Castellucci P, et al. FDG PET and 90Y ibritumomab tiuxetan in patients with follicular lymphoma. Q J Nucl Med Mol Imaging. 2010;54:436–41.

110. Jacene HA, Filice R, Kasecamp W, Wahl RL. 18 F-FDG PET/CT for monitoring the response of lymphoma to radioimmunotherapy. J Nucl Med. 2009;50:8–17.

111. Brunetti GA, Tendas A, Meloni E, et al. Pain and anxiety associated with bone marrow aspiration and biopsy: a prospective study on 152 Italian patients with hematological malignancies. Ann Hematol. 2011;90:1233–5.

112. Bain BJ. Morbidity associated with bone marrow aspiration and trephine biopsy: a review of UK data for 2004. Haematologica. 2006;91:1293–4.

113. Cheson BD, Fisher RI, Barrington SF, et al. Recommendations for initial evaluation, staging, and response assessment of Hodgkin and non-Hodgkin lymphoma: the Lugano classification. J Clin Oncol. 2014;32:3059–68.

114. El-Galaly TC, d'Amore F, Mylam KJ, et al. Routine bone marrow biopsy has little or no therapeutic consequence for positron emission tomography/computed tomography-staged treatment-naïve patients with Hodgkin lymphoma. J Clin Oncol. 2012;30:4508–14.

115. Khan AB, Barrington SF, Mikhaeel NG, et al. PET-CT staging of DLBCL accurately identifies and provides new insight into the clinical significance of bone marrow involvement. Blood. 2013;122:61–7.

116. Adams HJ, Kwee TC, de Keizer B, et al. FDG PET/CT for the detection of bone marrow involvement in diffuse large B-cell lymphoma: Systematic review and meta-analysis. Eur J Nucl Med Mol Imaging. 2014;41:565–74.

117. Adams HJ, Kwee TC, Fijnheer R, et al. Bone marrow 18 F-fluoro-2-deoxy-D-glucose positron emission tomography/computed tomography cannot replace bone marrow biopsy in diffuse large B-cell lymphoma. Am J Hematol. 2014;89:726–31.

118. Adams HJ, Kwee TC, Fijnheer R, et al. Direct comparison of visual and quantitative bone marrow FDG-PET/CT findings with bone marrow biopsy results in diffuse large B-cell lymphoma: does bone marrow FDG-PET/CT live up to its promise? Acta Radiol. 2015;56(10):1230–5.

119. Adams HJ, Kwee TC, Fijnheer R, et al. Utility of quantitative FDG-PET/CT for the detection of bone marrow involvement in follicular lymphoma: a histopathological correlation study. Skeletal Radiol. 2014;43:1231–6.

120. El-Najjar I, Montoto S, McDowell A, et al. The value of semiquantitative analysis in identifying diffuse bone marrow involvement in follicular lymphoma. Nucl Med Commun. 2014;35:311–5.

121. Adams HJ, Kwee TC, Fijnheer R, et al. Bone marrow FDG-PET/CT in Hodgkin lymphoma revisited: do imaging and pathology match? Ann Nucl Med. 2015;29:132–7.

122. Salaun PY, Gastinne T, Bodet-Milin C, et al. Analysis of 18F-FDG PET diffuse bone marrow uptake and splenic uptake in staging of Hodgkin's lymphoma: a reflection of disease infiltration or just inflammation? Eur J Nucl Med Mol Imaging. 2009;36:1813–21.

123. Bradley AJ, Carrington BM, Lawrance JA, et al. Assessment and significance of mediastinal bulk in Hodgkin's disease: comparison between computed tomography and chest radiography. J Clin Oncol. 1999;17:2493–8.

124. Gobbi PG, Ghirardelli ML, Solcia M, Di Giulio G, et al. Image-aided estimate of tumor burden in Hodgkin's disease: evidence of its primary prognostic importance. J Clin Oncol. 2001;19:1388–94.

125. Gobbi PG, Broglia C, Di Giulio G, et al. The clinical value of tumor burden at diagnosis in Hodgkin lymphoma. Cancer. 2004;101:1824–34.

126. Lister TA, Crowther D, Sutcliffe SB, et al. Report of a committee convened to discuss the evaluation and staging of patients with Hodgkin's disease: Cotswolds Meeting. J Clin Oncol. 1989;7:1630–6.

127. Hasenclever D, Diehl V. A prognostic score for advanced Hodgkin's disease: International Prognostic Factors Project on Advanced Hodgkin's Disease. N Engl J Med. 1998;339:1506–14.

128. Diehl V, Thomas RK, Re D. Part II: Hodgkin's lymphoma: diagnosis and treatment. Lancet Oncol. 2004;5:19–26.

129. Hoppe RT, Advani RH, Bierman PJ, et al. NCCN Hodgkin disease clinical practice guidelines in oncology. 2006 v.1. Available at: http://www.nccn.org. Last accessed 6 Jan 2006.

130. Song MK, Chung JS, Lee JJ, et al. Metabolic tumor volume by positron emission tomography/computed tomography as a clinical parameter to determine therapeutic modality for early stage Hodgkin's lymphoma. Cancer Sci. 2013;104:1656–61.

131. Kanoun S, Rossi C, Berriolo-Riedinger A, et al. Baseline metabolic tumour volume is an independent prognostic factor in Hodgkin lymphoma. Eur J Nucl Med Mol Imaging. 2014;41:1735–43.

132. Tseng D, Rachakonda LP, Su Z, et al. Interim-treatment quantitative PET parameters predict progression and death among patients with Hodgkin's disease. Radiat Oncol. 2012;7:5.

133. Hutchings M, Kostakoglu L, Zaucha JM, et al. In vivo treatment sensitivity testing with positron emission tomography/computed tomography after one cycle of chemotherapy for Hodgkin lymphoma. J Clin Oncol. 2014;32:2705–11.

134. Knight-Greenfield A, Cotter R, Marshall R, et al. Interim FDG PET/CT predicts response and progression free survival (PFS) better than baseline clinical and metabolic parameters in Hodgkin's lymphoma (HL): Correlation with various methodologies. J Nucl Med. 2013;54:69. Available at: http://jnm.snmjournals.org/content/54/supplement_2/69.abstract.

135. Federico M, Bellei M, Marcheselli L, et al. Follicular Lymphoma International Prognostic Index 2: a new prognostic index for follicular lymphoma developed by the International Follicular Lymphoma Prognostic Factor Project. J Clin Oncol. 2009;27:4555–62.

136. Pfreundschuh M, Ho AD, Cavallin-Stahl E, et al. Prognostic significance of maximum tumour (bulk) diameter in young adults with good-prognosis diffuse large-B-cell lymphoma treated with CHOP-like chemotherapy with or without rituximab: an exploratory analysis of the MabThera International Trial Group (MInT) study. Lancet Oncol. 2008;9:435–44.

137. Esfahani SA, Heidari P, Halpern EF, Hochberg EP, Palmer EL, Mahmood U. Baseline total lesion glycolysis measured with (18)F-FDG PET/CT as a predictor of progression-free survival in diffuse large B-cell lymphoma: a pilot study. Am J Nucl Med Mol Imaging. 2013;3:272–81.

138. Song MK, Chung JS, Shin HJ, Lee SM, Lee SE, Lee HS, Lee GW, Kim SJ, Lee SM, Chung DS. Clinical significance of metabolic tumor volume by PET/CT in stages II and III of diffuse large B cell lymphoma without extranodal site involvement. Ann Hematol. 2012;91:697–703.

139. Manohar K, Mittal BR, Bhattacharya A, Malhotra P, Varma S. Prognostic value of quantitative parameters derived on initial staging 18 F-fluorodeoxyglucose positron emission tomography/ computed tomography in patients with high-grade non-Hodgkin's lymphoma. Nucl Med Commun. 2012;33(9):974–81.

140. Sasanelli M, Meignan M, Haioun C, Berriolo-Riedinger A, Casasnovas RO, Biggi A, Gallamini A, Siegel BA, Cashen AF, Vera P, Tilly H, Versari A, Itti E. Pretherapy metabolic tumour volume is an independent predictor of outcome in patients with diffuse large B-cell lymphoma. Eur J Nucl Med Mol Imaging. 2014;41:2017–22.

141. Kim TM, Paeng JC, Chun IK, Keam B, Jeon YK, Lee SH, Kim DW, Lee DS, Kim CW, Chung JK, Kim IH, Heo DS. Total lesion glycolysis in positron emission tomography is a better predictor of outcome than the international prognostic index for patients with diffuse large B cell lymphoma. Cancer. 2013;119:1195–202.

142. Kim J, Hong J, Kim SG, et al. Prognostic value of metabolic tumor volume estimated by (18) F-FDG positron emission tomography/computed tomography in patients with diffuse large B-cell lymphoma of stage II or III disease. Nucl Med Mol Imaging. 2014;48:187–95.

143. Chihara D, Oki Y, Onoda H, et al. High maximum standard uptake value (SUVmax) on PET scan is associated with shorter survival in patients with diffuse large B cell lymphoma. Int J Hematol. 2011;93:502–8.

144. Xie M, Zhai W, Cheng S, Zhang H, Xie Y, He W. Predictive value of F-18 FDG PET/CT quantization parameters for progression-free survival in patients

with diffuse large B-cell lymphoma. Hematology. 2016;21(2):99–105.

145. Gallicchio R, Mansueto G, Simeon V, et al. F-18 FDG PET/CT quantization parameters as predictors of outcome in patients with diffuse large B-cell lymphoma. Eur J Haematol. 2014;92:382–9.

146. Adams HJ, de Klerk JM, Fijnheer R, et al. Prognostic superiority of the National Comprehensive Cancer Network International Prognostic Index over pre-treatment whole-body volumetric-metabolic FDG-PET/CT metrics in diffuse large B-cell lymphoma. Eur J Haematol. 2015;94:532–9.

147. Song MK, Chung JS, Shin HJ, et al. Prognostic value of metabolic tumor volume on PET / CT in primary gastrointestinal diffuse large B cell lymphoma. Cancer Sci. 2012;103:477–82.

148. Itti E, Meignan M, Berriolo-Riedinger A, et al. An international confirmatory study of the prognostic value of early PET/CT in diffuse large B-cell lymphoma: comparison between Deauville criteria and ΔSUVmax. Eur J Nucl Med Mol Imaging. 2013;40:1312–20.

149. Xie M, Wu K, Liu Y, Jiang Q, Xie Y. Predictive value of F-18 FDG PET/CT quantization parameters in diffuse large B cell lymphoma: a meta-analysis with 702 participants. Med Oncol. 2015;32:446.

150. Oh MY, Oh SB, Seoung HG, et al. Clinical significance of standardized uptake value and maximum tumor diameter in patients with primary extranodal diffuse large B cell lymphoma. Korean J Hematol. 2012;47:207–12.

151. Ceriani L, Martelli M, Zinzani PL, et al. Utility of baseline 18FDG-PET/CT functional parameters in defining prognosis of primary mediastinal (thymic) large B-cell lymphoma. Blood. 2015;126:950–6.

152. Lee PWD, Lavori P, Quon A, Hara W, Maxim P, Le QT, Wakelee H, Donington J, Graves E, Loo BW. Metabolic tumor burden predicts for disease progression and death in lung cancer. Int J Radiation Oncology Biol Phys. 2007;69:328–33.

153. Lin C, Itti E, Haioun C, et al. Early 18 F-FDG PET for prediction of prognosis in patients with diffuse large B-cell lymphoma: SUV-based assessment versus visual analysis. J Nucl Med. 2007;48:1626–32.

154. Itti E, Lin C, Dupuis J, et al. Prognostic value of interim 18 F-FDG PET in patients with diffuse large B-Cell lymphoma: SUV-based assessment at 4 cycles of chemotherapy. J Nucl Med. 2009;50:527–33.

155. Casasnovas RO, Meignan M, Berriolo-Riedinger A, et al. SUVmax reduction improves early prognosis value of interim positron emission tomography scans in diffuse large B-cell lymphoma. Blood. 2011;118:37–43.

156. Safar V, Dupuis J, Itti E, et al. Interim [18 F]fluoro-deoxyglucose positron emission tomography scan in diffuse large B-cell lymphoma treated with anthracycline-based chemotherapy plus rituximab. J Clin Oncol. 2012;30:184–90.

157. Nols N, Mounier N, Bouazza S, et al. Quantitative and qualitative analysis of metabolic response at interim positron emission tomography scan combined with International Prognostic Index is highly predictive of outcome in diffuse large B-cell lymphoma. Leuk Lymphoma. 2014;55:773–80.

158. Rossi C, Kanoun S, Berriolo-Riedinger A, et al. Interim 18 F-FDG PET SUVmax reduction is superior to visual analysis in predicting outcome early in Hodgkin lymphoma patients. J Nucl Med. 2014;55:569–73.

159. Gallamini A, Barrington SF, Biggi A, et al. The predictive role of interim Positron Emission Tomography on Hodgkin lymphoma treatment outcome is confirmed using the 5-point scale interpretation criteria. Haematologica. 2014;99:1107–13.

160. Biggi A, Gallamini A, Chauvie S, et al. International validation study for interim PET in ABVD-treated, advanced-stage Hodgkin lymphoma: interpretation criteria and concordance rate among reviewers. J Nucl Med. 2013;54:683–90.

161. Sharma P, Gupta A, Patel C, et al. Pediatric lymphoma: metabolic tumor burden as a quantitative index for treatment response evaluation. Ann Nucl Med. 2012;26:58–66.

162. Hussien AE, Furth C, Schönberger S, et al. FDG-PET response prediction in pediatric Hodgkin's lymphoma: impact of metabolically defined tumor volumes and individualized SUV measurements on the positive predictive value. Cancers (Basel). 2015;7:287–304.

163. Furth C, Steffen IG, Amthauer H, et al. Early and late therapy response assessment with [18 F]fluoro-deoxyglucose positron emission tomography in pediatric Hodgkin's lymphoma: analysis of a prospective multicenter trial. J Clin Oncol. 2009;27:4385–91.

164. Furth C, Meseck RM, Steffen IG, et al. SUV-measurements and patient-specific corrections in pediatric Hodgkin-lymphoma: is there a benefit for PPV in early response assessment by FDG-PET? Pediatr Blood Cancer. 2012;59:475–80.

165. Hasenclever D, Kurch L, Mauz-Körholz C, et al. qPET – a quantitative extension of the Deauville scale to assess response in interim FDG-PET scans in lymphoma. Eur J Nucl Med Mol Imaging. 2014;41:1301–8.

166. Park S, Moon SH, Park LC, et al. The impact of baseline and interim PET/CT parameters on clinical outcome in patients with diffuse large B cell lymphoma. Am J Hematol. 2012;87:937–40.

167. Malek E, Sendilnathan A, Yellu M, et al. Metabolic tumor volume on interim PET is a better predictor of outcome in diffuse large B-cell lymphoma than semi-quantitative methods. Blood Cancer J. 2015;5, e326.

168. Zhou Z, Sehn LH, Rademaker AW, et al. An enhanced International Prognostic Index (NCCN-IPI) for patients with diffuse large B-cell lymphoma treated in the rituximab era. Blood. 2014;123:837–42.

169. Furth C, Steffen IG, Erdrich AS, et al. Explorative analyses on the value of interim PET for prediction of response in pediatric and adolescent non-Hodgkin lymphoma patients. EJNMMI Res. 2013;3(1):71.

170. Tateishi U, Tatsumi M, Terauchi T, et al. Prognostic significance of metabolic tumor burden by positron emission tomography/computed tomography in patients with relapsed/refractory diffuse large B-cell lymphoma. Cancer Sci. 2015;106:186–93.

171. Walker AJ, Chirindel A, Hobbs RF, et al. Use of standardized uptake value thresholding for target volume delineation in pediatric Hodgkin lymphoma. Pract Radiat Oncol. 2015;5:219–27.

172. Vera P, Modzelewski R, Hapdey S, et al. Does enhanced CT influence the biological GTV measurement on FDG-PET images? Radiother Oncol. 2013;108:86–90.

173. Punwani S, Prakash V, Bainbridge A, et al. Quantitative diffusion weighted MRI: a functional biomarker of nodal disease in Hodgkin lymphoma? Cancer Biomark. 2010;7(4):249–59.

174. de Jong A, Kwee TC, de Klerk JM, et al. Relationship between pretreatment FDG-PET and diffusion-weighted MRI biomarkers in diffuse large B-cell lymphoma. Am J Nucl Med Mol Imaging. 2014;4: 231–8.

175. Hagtvedt T, Seierstad T, Lund KV, et al. Diffusion-weighted MRI compared to FDG PET/CT for assessment of early treatment response in lymphoma. Acta Radiol. 2015;56:152–8.

176. Mosavi F, Wassberg C, Selling J, Molin D, Ahlström H. Whole-body diffusion-weighted MRI and (18)F-FDG PET/CT can discriminate between different lymphoma subtypes. Clin Radiol. 2015;70:1229–36.

177. Usuda K, Maeda S, Motono N, et al. Diagnostic performance of diffusion – weighted imaging for multiple hilar and mediastinal lymph nodes with FDG accumulation. Asian Pac J Cancer Prev. 2015;16:6401–6.

178. Siegel MJ, Jokerst CE, Rajderkar D, et al. Diffusion-weighted MRI for staging and evaluation of response in diffuse large B-cell lymphoma: a pilot study. NMR Biomed. 2014;27:681–91.

179. Punwani S, Taylor SA, Saad ZZ, et al. Diffusion-weighted MRI of lymphoma: prognostic utility and implications for PET/MRI? Eur J Nucl Med Mol Imaging. 2013;40:373–85.

180. Trotman J, Luminari S, Boussetta S, et al. Prognostic value of PET-CT after first-line therapy in patients with follicular lymphoma: a pooled analysis of central scan review in three multicentre studies. Lancet Haematol. 2014;1:e17–27.

Amanda J. Walker and Stephanie A. Terezakis

5.1 History of Radiation Therapy in Hodgkin's Lymphoma

Only seven years after Wilhelm Conrad Röntgen discovered X-rays in 1895, the first documented case of Hodgkin's lymphoma (HL) was treated with radiotherapy [40]. William Allen Pusey, a professor of dermatology at the University of Illinois, had been using X-rays to treat a variety of dermatologic conditions. A 4-year-old boy with enlarged cervical lymph nodes "the size of a fist" was referred to Dr. Pusey and after irradiation the mass remarkably diminished to the size of an almond. In an era when there were no successful cancer therapies, 40 years before the

introduction of chemotherapy, Dr. Pusey and colleagues marveled at this seemingly magical response. Radiation was offered to subsequent patients with HL over the next few years, and although a response to therapy was almost always demonstrated, the treatment was palliative. Primitive treatment machines were only capable of delivering low energy X-rays and the disease inevitably recurred.

In the early 1920s, kilovoltage equipment was developed. This allowed higher doses of radiation therapy to penetrate deeper into tissue with more skin-sparing effects. René Gilbert, a Swiss radiologist, was the first to report durable responses in treating patients with HL using kV X-rays with larger treatment fields that also included lymph node regions that were not obviously involved with disease. A number of patients treated in this way had a remarkable long-term survival [15], and by the 1950s, Vera Peters at the Ontario Institute of Radiotherapy had studied enough patients to report that early-stage HL can be cured with fractionated radiation therapy using large fields [39]. By the 1970s it had been established that the standard of care for early-stage HL was RT with fields aimed at all of the clinically relevant lymph node regions of the body [25]. Around this time, outcomes for advanced disease were further improved with the introduction of multi-agent chemotherapy regimens [11]. Radiation remains one of the most effective modalities for the treatment of HL as lymphomas and

A.J. Walker, MD
Department of Radiation Oncology and Molecular Radiation Sciences, Johns Hopkins University School of Medicine and Sidney Kimmel Comprehensive Cancer Center, Baltimore, MD, USA

S.A. Terezakis, MD (✉)
Department of Radiation Oncology and Molecular Radiation Sciences, Johns Hopkins University School of Medicine and Sidney Kimmel Comprehensive Cancer Center, Baltimore, MD, USA

Department of Radiation Oncology & Molecular Radiation Sciences, Sidney Kimmel Comprehensive Cancer Center, 401 N. Broadway, Suite 1440, Baltimore, MD 21287, USA
e-mail: stereza1@jhmi.edu

© Springer International Publishing Switzerland 2016
A. Gallamini (ed.), *PET Scan in Hodgkin Lymphoma*, DOI 10.1007/978-3-319-31797-7_5

lymphatic tissue in general are highly radiosensitive. It is well known that the sensitivity of cells to radiation is proportional to the degree of proliferative activity and inversely proportional to the degree of differentiation. In other words, undifferentiated cells with high mitotic capability, such as the cells within malignant nodes in HL, are more likely to be radiosensitive. Of course, other factors play a role, including the oxygen concentration (hypoxic tumors are less sensitive to radiation) and inherent cellular response to DNA damage.

Over the last 40 years, radiation delivery techniques have continued to improve. This allowed for a more uniform dose distribution and better-targeted therapy. Advances were seen in other disciplines as well – more effective and less toxic multi-agent chemotherapy agents were developed, there were vast improvements in radiographic imaging, we obtained a better understanding of prognostic factors, and after rigorous study we made strides toward tailoring therapy based on stage and risk classification. In the modern era, early-stage HL is commonly treated with combined chemotherapy and radiation. Advanced disease is generally treated with more intensive chemotherapy regimens, while RT is reserved for bulky masses or areas of residual disease after chemotherapy. Today with combined modality treatment, HL has one of the highest cure rates of all malignancies with long-term survival over 80 %.

Unfortunately these high cure rates have come with a price. The majority of HL patients are children or young adults and late effects of treatment can be devastating and has an impact on survival. Two of the most significant late effects include development of secondary malignancy and cardiovascular disease [1, 3, 6]. It is felt that the risk of developing a radiation-induced secondary malignancy is related to both dose and field size. In a retrospective study of patients treated for HL, death caused by heart disease was exceeded only by death caused by HL and other neoplasms. Mediastinal irradiation increases the risk of subsequent death from heart disease, and this risk increases with total dose delivered to the mediastinum, minimal cardiac blocking, and young age at treatment [21].

Radiation continues to have an important role in ensuring locoregional control and improving overall outcome in the combined modality treatment approach for HL, but efforts have been made to minimize treatment judiciously in order to lower the impact of late effects on morbidity and mortality. One of the most dramatic ways in which we have scaled back treatment has been the reduction in radiation field size as we move away from elective nodal irradiation with involved field radiation to more targeted conformal approaches with involved-node and involved-site radiotherapy. Central to this paradigm shift have been improvements in radiation delivery techniques, including the incorporation of FDG-PET/CT into the design of radiation treatment fields.

Although multiple radiopharmaceuticals exist, ^{18}F-FDG is the most widely available and widely used radiopharmaceutical in oncology including in HL. Therefore ^{18}F-FDG will be the focus of this text. PET/CT has proven its value in staging for HL as well as in evaluating treatment response and has been increasingly used as an imaging method for the planning of radiation therapy for lymphomas.

5.2   Evolution of Radiation Treatment Fields

Historically lymphoma was managed with extended fields that encompassed all of the lymph node regions in the body, given the possibility of microscopic extension of disease outside the areas of palpable disease as well as reports of distant recurrences after local radiotherapy alone. These traditional extended fields are illustrated in Fig. 5.1. A mantle field includes the lymph node regions above the diaphragm and the inverted-Y field includes the lymph node regions in the abdomen and pelvis. When an inverted-Y field was combined with mantle field radiation, the combination was referred to as *total nodal irra-*

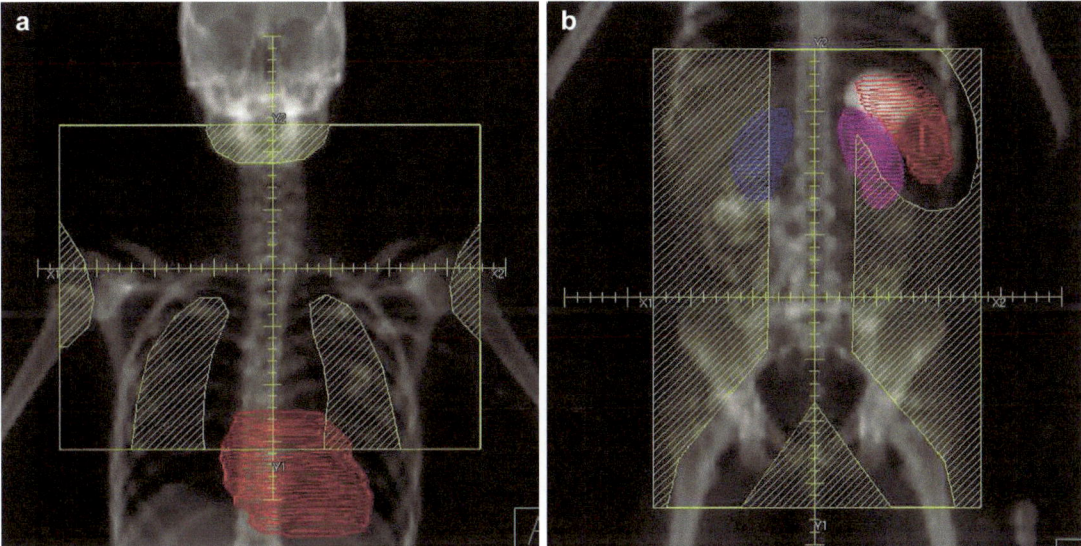

Fig. 5.1 Historical radiation fields. Digitally reconstructed radiographs of (**a**) mantle and (**b**) inverted-Y extended fields

diation. At the time, single-modality radiation was preferred over the mechlorethamine, vincristine (Oncovin), procarbazine, and prednisone (MOPP) regimen of chemotherapy given its high rates of sterility and secondary leukemia, and chemotherapy was reserved for cases of disease refractory to RT. Radiation was delivered with linear accelerators using two-dimensional planning. 2-D planning makes use of an X-ray simulator and a two-dimensional treatment planning system used for calculation of dose distribution after the radiation oncologist defines treatment fields based on bony anatomy.

In the 1980s, computerized tomography (CT) revolutionized the imaging of tumors. CT scans were not only helpful for the radiation oncologist because they allowed for a better understanding of the tumor and normal tissue in 3-dimensions, but by the 1990s, CTs also became a critical component of treatment planning and a routine part of cancer management. An additional advantage of CT scan for radiation planning is that Hounsfield units (metrics to quantify tissue radiodensity) are correlated with electron density of tissue at each voxel relative to the electron density of water. Due to this correlation it became possible to use

information from the CT to calculate radiation absorption and scattering in tissue. In the modern era of 3-D planning, the radiation oncologist contours the volume of tissue to be irradiated as well as normal structures. Dose parameters can then be calculated for any region that is contoured on the planning software. In this process of contouring, the radiation oncologist utilizes all available information regarding the patient's anatomy, including diagnostic CT, MRI, PET, ultrasound, physical exam, as well as reports from any endoscopic procedures or operations. Using the treatment planning software, it is possible to fuse other imaging modalities to the planning CT such that information from both PET and MRI can be seamlessly incorporated into target volume delineation on the planning CT. In this way, the PET is directly incorporated into the process of radiation treatment planning.

In the 1990s and early 2000s, it was recognized that when chemotherapy was added to radiation therapy, the extended field could be replaced with a smaller field known as the "involved field," which remained the standard of care until recently [49]. Involved field radiation encompasses not only the involved lymph nodes but also the other lymph nodes within the same lymph node region defined by the Ann Arbor classification for HL staging. All of the field borders were based on bony landmarks such that they could be planned on 2-D simulation units.

A review of relapses in patients treated with chemotherapy alone showed that most recurrences occur in the initially involved lymph nodes [42]. With continued advances in radiation technology and imaging, including 3-D planning and the introduction of FDG-PET scans, it became possible to further minimize treatment fields to only include the initially involved nodal volume in an effort to minimize radiation dose to normal tissues. This concept was introduced in 2006 by the EORTC-GELA in the form of involved nodal radiation therapy (INRT) [18].

Unlike the involved field, which included adjacent uninvolved lymph nodes, INRT limited treatment to only the pre and post-chemotherapy involved lymph node remnant(s) plus a relatively small margin for setup error of 1 cm [18]. The shift from involved field to involved-node radiation techniques mirrored the larger shift within the field of radiation oncology from 2D planning based on bony landmarks and more conformal radiation delivery with 3D treatment planning using CT scans. For the first time, ICRU (International Commission on Radiation Units and Measurements) terms were formally incorporated into the management of HL. These terms include the gross tumor volume (GTV), clinical target volume (CTV), and planning target volume (PTV). GTV refers to the position and extent of gross tumor, i.e., what can be seen, palpated, or imaged. The CTV contains the GTV plus a margin for sub-clinical disease spread. This is often the most difficult volume to contour because this area cannot be fully imaged and it is difficult to accurately define. The PTV includes the CTV plus a margin to account for setup uncertainty. The PTV is the volume to which an isodose line is prescribed. In order to successfully implement INRT, patients must have pre- and post-chemotherapy contrast-enhanced CT scans in the treatment position, and whenever possible the pretreatment CT is performed in conjunction with a PET/CT, also in the treatment position. A major advantage of incorporating the PET/CT into RT planning for INRT is that it can identify previously undetected lymph nodes that are likely to contain disease. As initially involved lymph nodes are usually either no longer visible or of normal size, a CTV is contoured that is the initial location and extent of disease prior to chemotherapy. Per the EORTC-GELA INRT guidelines, a 1 cm isotropic margin around the CTV was recommended as the PTV in most situations to account for internal organ motion and setup error [17]. Examples of IFRT and INRT treatment fields are also shown in Fig. 5.2.

Because INRT requires precisely fused pre- and post-chemotherapy images (including PET/CT) in the treatment position, the International Lymphoma Radiation Oncology Group (ILROG) introduced the concept of Involved Site Radiation Therapy (ISRT) in 2013 [44]. One of the differences between ISRT and INRT is related to the quality and accuracy (i.e., patient positioning) of the pre-chemotherapy imaging. ISRT incorporates the opportunity to create larger CTV volumes associated with uncertainties related to less than optimal pretreatment imaging (e.g., the pretreatment PET/CT is not obtained in the treatment position). Per the ISRT guidelines, it is recommended that when contouring the CTV, one takes into account the quality and accuracy of imaging, volume changes since imaging, any potential disease spread, potential subclinical involvement, and adjacent normal tissue. There remains a great deal of subjectivity to this process and quantitative imaging, such as PET/CT can be an invaluable tool in order to minimize this inter-observer variability. The approach to ISRT planning is shown in Fig. 5.3.

Both INRT and ISRT would not be possible without the many advances in the field of radiation therapy over the past two decades including computer-assisted 3D planning and treatment delivery. More precise delivery of radiation is now possible with maximum coverage of target volumes and more normal tissue sparing due to the development of intensity-modulated radiotherapy (IMRT) and 3D conformal RT. Technical advances with dynamic multi-leaf collimators, image-guided radiation therapy, and improve-

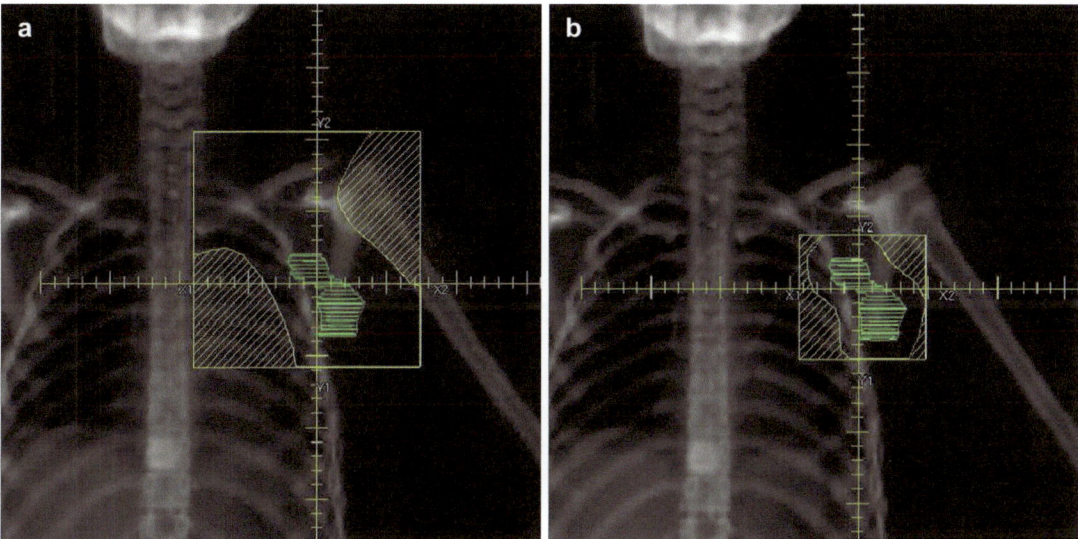

Fig. 5.2 Axillary radiation fields with (**a**) IFRT and (**b**) INRT displayed on digitally reconstructed radiographs. The volume contoured in green encompasses the pre-chemotherapy GTV. This volume represents the CTV in INRT treatment planning. In IFRT, the axillary field includes ipsilateral infraclavicular and supraclavicular lymph node regions with the superior extent of the field at C5–C6 interspace

ments in patient immobilization and positioning all facilitate the delivery of highly complex, multi-field, conformal treatment plans. In order to take full advantage of the recent and dramatic advances in radiation treatment delivery methods and successfully implement INRT/ISRT, the most accurate and precise target delineation is required. In the pre-PET era, the definitions of tumor volumes and treatment volumes were based primarily on structural imaging with contrast CT, physical exam findings, and clinical judgment. The clinical target volume represents the microscopic extent of disease. Although there is no way to image the CTV directly, it is formed with a margin applied to the GTV that was contoured on the pretreatment planning CT and in most cases fused to the pretreatment PET/CT adjusting for changes in the position of normal tissues. Microscopic disease may be missed if the imaging fails to precisely define the extent of tumor. Additionally, further reduction in field size necessitates increased precision, and thus, the value of PET/CT for the planning of ISRT has dramatically increased. Although there is no data to suggest that incorporating PET/CT into volumes leads to improvement in disease related

outcomes, it is viewed as an invaluable resource and the incorporation of PET/CT into RT treatment planning has become a central component of modern HL therapy with INRT and ISRT.

5.3   Impact of PET on Target Volume Delineation in Hodgkin's Lymphoma

As discussed in Chap. 1, there is a higher accuracy in HL staging with FDG-PET scan, compared to CT alone. Furthermore, studies in lymphoma as well as other malignancies have shown that the estimate of tumor extent is more accurate when functional and structural images are combined (see Chapter 4). Functional imaging with PET can influence RT planning for HL in a number of ways. PET can reveal areas of disease that are not well visualized by other imaging modalities. These areas represent additional areas of disease adjacent to the primary tumor volume or unsuspected lymph nodes (LN) or extranodal sites (ENS) involved with disease. Moreover, upon PET/CT incorporation, equivocally involved LN or ENS on CT or MRI, benign reac-

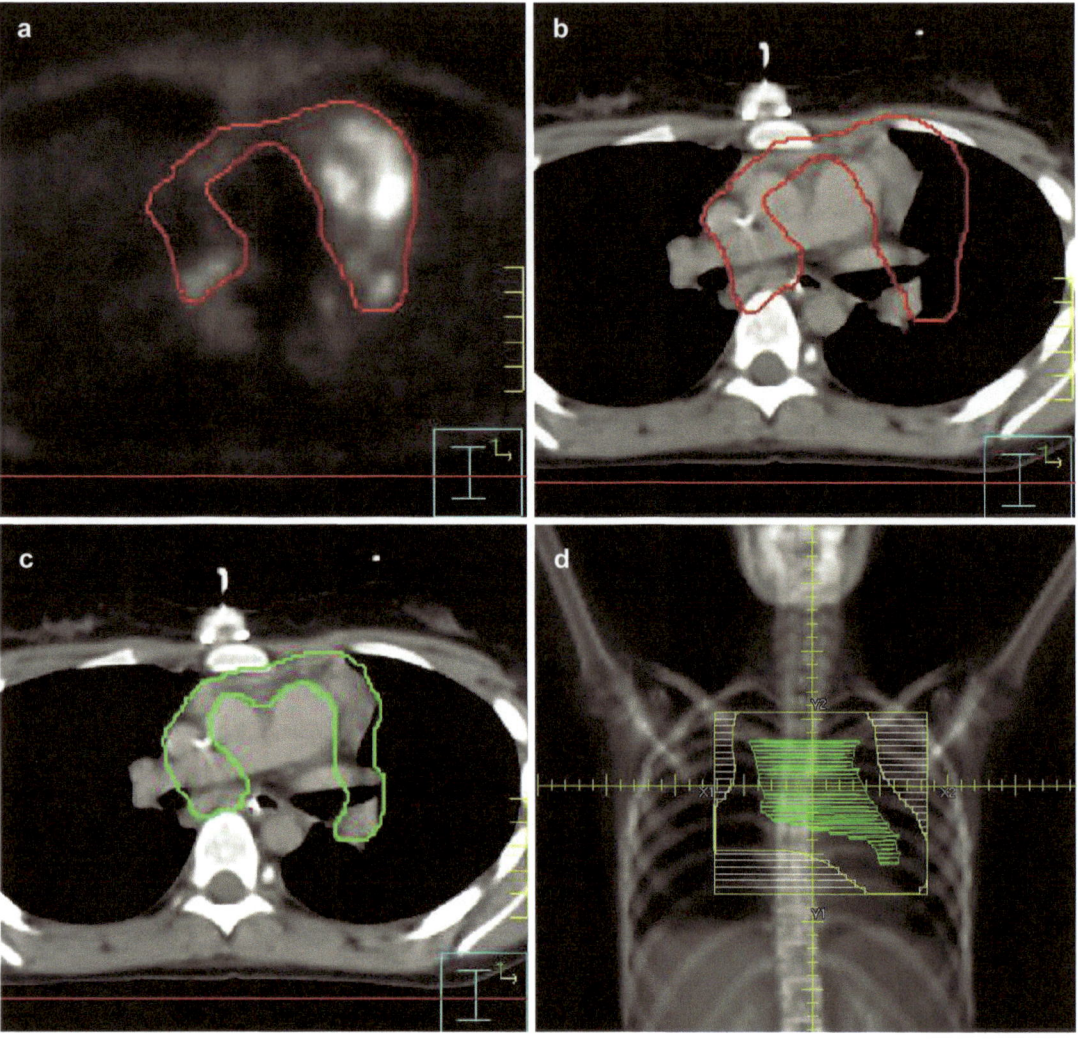

Fig. 5.3 Involved-site radiation therapy (ISRT). (**a**) Pre-chemotherapy GTV based on PET/CT. (**b**) Pre-chemotherapy GTV on post-chemotherapy planning CT. (**c**) Clinical target volume encompassing the extent of ini-tial disease, created by modifying the pre-chemotherapy GTV on post-chemotherapy planning CT. (**d**) Digitally reconstructed radiograph of AP field

tive lymphadenopathy or brown fat tissue will be less likely included in the radiation field. As discussed in Chap. 2, PET is also useful in evaluating residual masses after chemotherapy and can aid in the final decision regarding radiation dose in HL since higher doses are required for macroscopic compared to microscopic disease.

As mentioned above, there have yet to be randomized prospective studies to demonstrate an improvement in clinical outcome combining both imaging techniques for RT planning compared to CT alone, since FDG-PET has been widely adopted together with CT into routine standard practice. However, the impact of FDG-PET in radiation planning for HL has been addressed in a number of studies, which are summarized in Table 5.1. The proportion of HL cases in which there are changes in target volume with the incorporation of PET into RT planning in these studies ranges from 17 to 70%. In general, FDG-PET is more likely to increase rather than decrease treatment field size, and significant changes in the

Table 5.1 Studies addressing the impact of FDG-PET on radiation planning

Study	RT field	No. of pts	Median age (range)	Histology	Findings with addition of PET to treatment planning
Hutchings 2007	IFRT	30	35 (18–79)	HL	10 patients (33 %) had change in field size 7 patients (23 %) had increase in treatment volume 2 patients (6 %) had decrease in treatment volume 1 patient had upstaging from IIB to IIIBS based on splenic involvement
Girinsky 2007	INRT	30	Not reported	HL	36 % of patients had increase in field size PET increased average target volume to 313 cm³ from 291 cm³ without PET; $p = 0.0007$
Paulino 2011	IFRT	53	14 (6–21)	HL	9 patients (17 %) had change in field size 8 patients (15 %) had increase in treatment volume 1 patient (2 %) had decrease in treatment volume
Robertson 2011	IFRT	30	14 (5–18)	HL	21 patients (70 %) had change in field size 32 sites were added and 15 sites were excluded
Terezakis 2011	IFRT	29	58 (21–88)	5 HL 21 NHL 3 plasma cell	23 treatment sites (72 %) had change in field size 15 sites (47 %) had increase in treatment volume (median 11 % increase) 8 sites (25 %) had decrease in treatment volume (median of 20 % decrease)

radiation field tend to occur with the incorporation of FDG-avid lymph nodes that would not have been included with CT planning alone. This is critical in the application of INRT and ISRT where the potential for a marginal miss is enhanced. Reasons for the difference in reported changes may be due to the different methods for defining the RT field, different inclusion criteria (e.g., age) and the fields that were evaluated (e.g., supradiaphragmatic disease only vs. supra- and infradiaphragmatic fields).

In 2004 Lee et al. reported one of the earliest studies addressing the feasibility and impact of incorporating PET into RT treatment fields in lymphoma [30]. Seventeen PET scans from patients with thoracic lymphoma (both HL and NHL) were registered to CT. Comparisons were made between GTV on PET compared to GTV on CT in regard to total volume, as well as lateral and inferior extension of the volume. Of note, the authors did not include both CT and PET information in delineating GTV, as is often done in modern treatment planning. Of the patients who had disease visible on both imaging techniques, the median total CT volume was larger than the total PET volume. In drawing lateral blocks, there were differences >3.0 cm in 40 % of cases. In only three cases the GTV based on PET was smaller than the GTV based on CT. Furthermore, the inferior CT extent of disease was in general lower to that of PET. Although contouring with PET led to significant differences in GTV extent compared to CT alone, the treatment fields were only minimally impacted since conformal treatment methods were not used. The authors conclude that incorporating PET into treatment planning is feasible and the influence of PET in thoracic lymphoma radiation fields appears to be modest.

The subsequent studies examining the impact of PET/CT in RT field design using IFRT or INRT including areas outside of the mediastinum did not agree with this conclusion. Hutchings et al. retrospectively evaluated the treatment plans for 30 adult patients with early-stage HL who underwent PET/CT prior to chemotherapy with adriamycin, bleomycin, vinblastine, dacarbazine (ABVD) [23]. They each received IFRT as defined by the Nordic guidelines after chemotherapy. The radiation oncologists were blinded on the PET result; therefore only CT was used in the treatment field delineation. According to the Nordic guidelines, the radiation field according to IFRT modality encompasses only the tissue volume that had contained the anatomical extent of detectable HL masses prior to chemotherapy, with an additional margin of at least 3 cm while sparing the remaining Ann Arbor lymph node region uninvolved by disease. In this study, the patients received 30.6 Gy in 1.8 Gy daily fractions with a boost of 5.4 Gy to areas of residual disease after chemotherapy. After completion of the RT course, the delineation of treatment fields was repeated on the planning CT scan including information from staging PET CT images. The study was aimed at assessing the contribution of PET/CT to a CT-defined radiation volume; a radiologist and a nuclear medicine expert delineated the radiation field in CT and PET, respectively. When a focus was defined as PET positive, the actual delineation of the target volume was performed using the corresponding CT images for the precise anatomical definition and target volumes defined based on the Nordic IFRT guidelines. In 10 of the 30 patients (approximate 33 %), the delineation of the CTV would have been changed by PET/CT. Seven patients had sites of PET involvement that were outside of the irradiated volume; hence the final irradiated volume would have increased. In these patients, the volume receiving a minimum of 90 % of the prescribed dose was increased by 8–87 % (median

17 %). In two patients, PET CT would have decreased the irradiated volume, and the volume receiving a minimum of 90 % of the prescribed dose was decreased by 18 % and 30 %. One patient had evidence of FDG uptake in the spleen that had not been visible on CT and was upstaged from stage IIB to stage IIIBS. Given that the majority of patients had an increase in treatment field size, it was recommended that FDG-PET should be used to reduce the amount of tissue receiving radiation therapy and would be warranted in RT planning for smaller fields such as INRT. It is noteworthy that of the 30 patients who received IFRT based on CT only in this study, 29 are in complete remission at the time of publication after a median follow-up of 24 months. One patient relapsed within the irradiated field after 2.8 years in a site that was positive on both CT and PET.

Robertson et al. performed a similar study in the pediatric HL population [41]. A nuclear medicine physician experienced in pediatric PET imaging interpreted the staging PET/CT. IFRT was delivered with a CTV created that covered that particular anatomic region as defined by the Ann Arbor staging system. The methods were slightly different in that all relevant lymph node sites and extranodal sites were systematically evaluated in 30 patients and analyzed separately by both CT and FDG-PET. Criteria for anatomic and functional imaging were defined by the current Children's Oncology Group (COG) protocol guidelines. The CT criteria were based on lymph node size depending on anatomical location. The PET criteria, on the other hand, remained rather subjective with "the level of tumor uptake assessed subjectively by visual inspection and semi-quantitatively by determination of SUV." The authors found an overall 14 % discordant rate between PET and CT results with more disagreement in nodal vs. extranodal sites. When the studies disagreed for a particular anatomic location, it was more common for the PET to be positive with a negative CT than vice versa. Thirty-two new sites were added and 15 sites were excluded from the IFRT fields, which altered the final treatment volumes in an impressive 21 of 30 (70 %) of patients. The most commonly added sites were the contralateral neck, para-aortic nodes, and spleen. The most commonly excluded sites were pleura, pericardia, and lung nodules. The authors concluded that PET was particularly helpful in detecting disease in relatively small lymph nodes in the neck and axilla that were below CT size criteria and was also superior in revealing disease in areas that are difficult to visualize on CT such as in the abdomen near the head of the pancreas. Patients in this study were treated to 21 Gy in either 1.5 or 1.8 Gy fractions. Four of the 30 (13 %) had relapsed at some point during or after treatment. There were no recurrences in sites excluded from RT based on PET with the exception of an axillary recurrence in a node that was not considered FDG avid nor positive on CT and therefore was not included in the treatment field. In retrospect, however, the site was reinterpreted as hypermetabolic at time of initial staging highlighting the importance of identifying initially involved lymph nodes for RT field delineation. The other three recurrences were within RT treatment fields in areas that were positive on CT and PET.

Paulino et al. also examined the impact of PET/CT on IFRT field design for pediatric HL. This was the largest cohort with 53 patients studied [38]. On CT scan, any node was considered involved with lymphoma if the transverse diameter was >1.5 cm above the diaphragm and >1 cm below the diaphragm (except mesenteric nodes where >1.5 cm was the cutoff). Staging PET CT was also performed where the level of tumor uptake was assessed subjectively by "visual inspection by a nuclear medicine physician and semi-quantitatively by determination of SUV" per COG guidelines. IFRT was delivered (21 Gy in 14 fractions) to all sites of initial disease plus the entire nodal region. IFRT fields were drawn with and without PET CT information and compared. According to the study design, in cases where there was a discrepancy between CT and PET/CT staging, sites of disease were confirmed by either biopsy ($n=4$) or by response to chemotherapy ($n=19$) prior to administering RT. On retrospective review, 19 of 53 patients (35.8 %) had discordance in at least 1 site between CT and PET/CT findings, which led to a

change in radiotherapy field in 9 (17 %). Upon PET/CT staging, the fields increased in size in 8 patients and decreased in 1, with a similar pattern reported in Hutchings et al. and Robertson et al. The most notable change in the RT field was the inclusion of the spleen in 4 cases. Twenty-five nodal sites and disease regions were examined, the specificity, sensitivity, and positive predictive value of PET being 99.5 %, 96.3 %, and 97.9 %, respectively, similar to that reported in previously published reports [13]. The author's conclusion was similar to that of Hutchings et al. that upon inclusion of PET/CT for IFRT planning, the size of radiation fields likely increases, a concept in sharp contrast to the ongoing paradigm shift toward decreasing treatment intensity (and therefore field size) to minimize late effects.

The relationship between PET/CT-aided RT planning and size of radiation fields was also addressed by Girinsky et al. [16]. Thirty patients with early-stage HL who were treated with INRT according to the EORTC-GELA guidelines were included in the study. All tumor masses but one were FDG-avid prior to chemotherapy. FDG helped localize undetected lymph nodes on CT scan in 36 % of the patients and the metabolic information from pre-chemotherapy PET/CT significantly modified the final irradiation volumes – the average volume incorporating PET was 313 cm^3 (95 % CI: 230–397) compared to 291 cm^3 by CT (95 % CI: 212–370) ($p=0.0007$). In this study, the only recurrence after a median of 2 years was in an unirradiated area in a patient with stage II disease treated with ABVD.

Terezakis et al. report similar results in the examination of patients with HL, NHL, and plasma cell neoplasms [46]. They found that with the incorporation of PET in the definition of IFRT fields, treatment volume had increased in 15 sites (47 %) by a median of 11 % and treatment volume was reduced in 8 sites (25 %) by a median of 20 %.

Despite the limitations of these studies, including the retrospective nature of the analysis, lack of statistical validation due to small sample size, and mainly descriptive methods applicable to this type of data, each provides valuable insight into the role of PET/CT in treatment planning for HL. With the exception of Lee et al., which examined less modern treatment and imaging techniques, these studies concordantly conclude that FDG-PET significantly changes the final treatment volumes in IFRT and INRT fields. Moreover, the incorporation of PET is recommended for modern conformal fields such as INRT and ISRT, as is the current treatment paradigm.

5.4 Methods for Incorporating FDG-PET in RT Planning

After co-registration of the pretreatment PET/CT to the posttreatment planning CT, the target volume should be delineated as described above. Ideally, only the tumor-dependent FDG uptake should be included in the radiation field, while the unspecific FDG uptake by inflammatory tissue should not be taken into account. Prior to the introduction of PET/CT, the definition of an involved lymph node in HL was variable. The dimensional criteria, with a threshold of 1–1.5 cm in the longest transverse diameter as suggestive of lymphoma harbinger, were generally accepted [7]. There are many objections to this definition including a technical limitation related to the fact that cross-sectional lymph node dimension may vary in different spatial directions on CT scan, lymph node architecture can be modified by tumor invasion, and, most importantly, lymph nodes can contain disease without a significant increase in size. An additional layer of complexity is added due to inter-observer variability with CT scanning.

The EORTC-GELA guidelines on how to incorporate PET CT into treatment planning for INRT are summarized below [17].

- Both planning CT and PET/CT images in the treatment position must be obtained prior to chemotherapy and planning CT images only after chemotherapy. All images should be contrast-enhanced.
- Pre-chemotherapy PET/CT should be carefully analyzed to identify any lymph nodes that may have been overlooked on CT. An

example of an FDG-avid lymph node overlooked on CT is shown in Fig. 5.4.
- Comparison of pre- and post-chemo images, both for morphologic asymmetry on CT and functional asymmetry on PET/CT, can be an indicator of disease involvement (e.g., involved lymph nodes may decrease in size or disappear entirely).

With the movement from extended field to involved field and more recently to involved-node or involved-site radiotherapy, there has been a strong desire to generate more specific guidelines on target volume delineation including how to interpret imaging results from the PET/CT scan, particularly given the degree of inter-observer variability. As it stands, no consensus has emerged.

5.4.1 Automated and Semi-automated Methods of Target Volume Definition

All of the studies and guidelines mentioned thus far have focused around using a primarily qualitative visual assessment of FDG-PET to aid in target delineation. This inherently subjective method requires input from an experienced radiologist and/or nuclear medicine physician and is prone to inter- and intra-observer variability. Contouring the tumor with the aid of PET is particularly prone to variability as one can easily make the GTV appear larger or smaller on the PET scan by adjusting the threshold levels in the planning or image viewing software. Despite these limitations, the visual interpretation method reflects the current level of practice.

One challenge with PET imaging in particular is the issue of edge detection. The appearance of the lesion edge on PET can by influenced by a number of factors related to the size and shape of the lesion. One way to address this problem is to fuse the PET with cross-sectional anatomy on CT scan as is often done in clinical practice. The edges that are not well defined on PET may be better defined on CT. However, in areas of disease that are imbedded within an area of similar Hounsfield units (e.g., tumor next to atelectatic

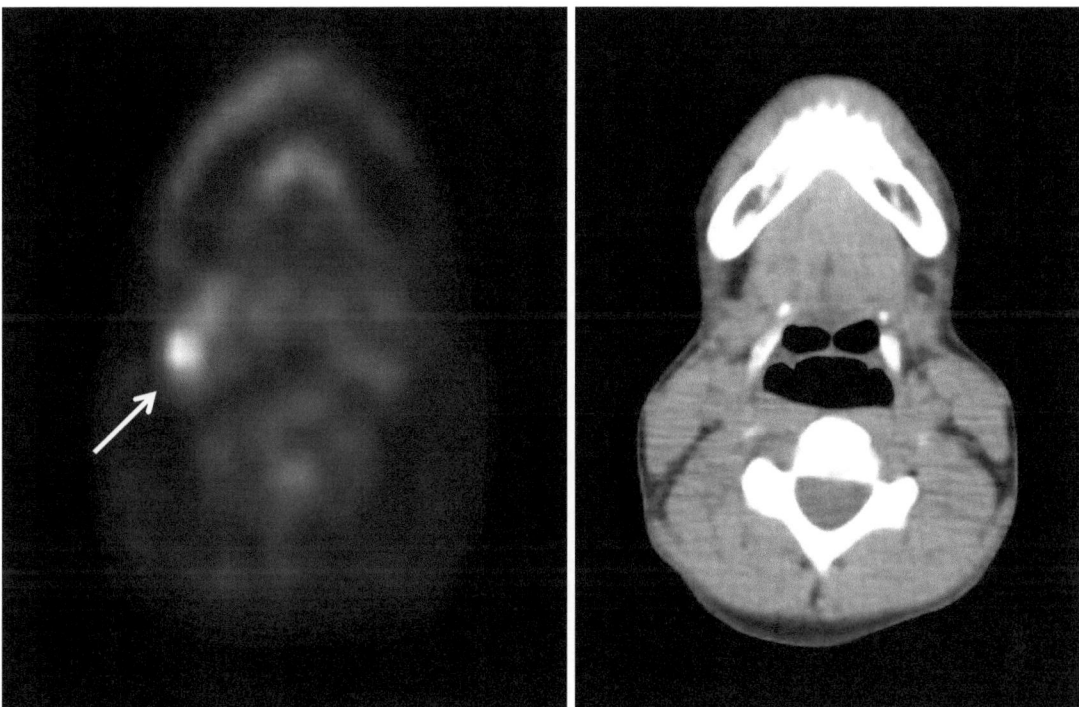

Fig. 5.4 FDG-avid lymph node in right cervical region that was overlooked on CT (*arrow*)

lung), this is not very helpful. Visual contouring is the most common method of defining edges in 3-dimensional space, but this again invites inter-observer variability and creates potential pitfalls with quality assurance.

Much controversy surrounds the value of PET in *tumor* volume delineation or the delineation of the pre-chemo GTV, which if performed in an automated or semiautomated way would require both a cutoff value and edge detection method-ologies. Those who do not believe that PET should be used to delineate tumor volumes base their argument on the fact that PET and CT are conceptually different imaging modalities [16]. Additionally, CT scan can provide an instanta-neous image, particularly when breath-hold tech-niques are utilized, and inherent in its nature, a PET scan produces an image over time and as a result cannot be controlled for motion (e.g., mediastinal mass motion during the breathing cycle). Spatial resolution is also different between the two and image windowing can dramatically change the size of a tumor mass on FDG-

PET. Regardless, PET remains an invaluable tool for target delineation given the metabolic infor-mation it provides that complements the ana-tomic information from CT scan [20].

Because PET is critical to implementing INRT and ISRT, some authors have suggested that a threshold-based target volume could be deter-mined in order to facilitate reproducibility from patient to patient and from physician to physician [29]. PET is a quantitative imaging technique; therefore mathematical models and imaging pro-cessing methods have been proposed to aid in contouring a PET volume using an automatic or semiautomatic methodology. All methods have advantages and disadvantages, and none have proven to be clearly superior to the others. However, it must always be remembered that in their current state, automated methods have a shared inherent weakness in that they cannot dif-ferentiate between FDG uptake due to malignancy compared to other benign conditions, which some would argue is the most challenging aspect of tar-get delineation with PET in radiation planning for lymphoma. A few of the most common automated and semiautomated methods of target volume delineation will be described below.

5.4.2 SUV

PET was ultimately developed as a quantitative tool. Although many methods have been developed [19], the SUV, despite its limitations, is the most widely used method for quantifying FDG-PET studies. In fact, most automatic or semiautomatic contouring methods involve SUV in some way. The SUV represents the FDG uptake within a tissue measured over a certain interval after FDG administration and normalized to the injected dose and to a factor that takes into account the distribution of FDG throughout the body (such as body weight) [28]. The determination of max SUV in a given lesion is a very common and reliable way to differentiate between benign and malignant conditions. However, one must always keep in mind that SUV should not be taken out of context, and absolute SUV measurements can be unreliable since it is a value that is affected by many factors. Technical factors such as errors in calibration between the PET scanner and dose calibrator [14], biologic factors such as patient comfort [2], and physical factors such as various image reconstruction parameters and region of interest (ROI) definitions [4] all play a role in SUV determination (see Chapter 4). It is also important to remember that a PET scan is not a sophisticated cancer map; it is simply a measure of glucose uptake in tissue. There are many other reasons why tissues take up glucose – e.g., physiologic reasons, inflammation, etc. which will be explained in more detail later in the chapter and more extensively in the Chap. 6 of this book.

5.4.3 Thresholding

The simplest method of using PET for target volume delineation is to use SUV itself. For example, in NSCLC, an SUV value ≥ 2.5 is considered abnormal and highly suspicious for tumor [22]. Although this approach may be reasonable for lung tumors, the appropriate SUV value cutoff is less clear for other malignancies such as head and neck cancer, esophageal cancer, and lymphoma. Furthermore, it is well known that benign conditions can lead to SUV >2.5 and small lesions and edges of moving lesions may falsely lower the SUV to <2.5 due to what is known as the partial volume effect.

Using an absolute threshold or cutoff value with SUV is not only helpful in determining which lesions represent disease, it is also a straightforward way to perform auto-segmentation (i.e., auto-contouring) [50]. In fact, one of the most common methods of contouring a tumor based on FDG-PET is using a fixed threshold method. For example, with a threshold cutoff value of 2.5, any voxel with an SUV of 2.5 or higher would be included the target volume.

In a similar way, a percent threshold for SUV_{max} or SUV_{peak} can be used instead of an absolute threshold value. In this method, the volume defined as tumor represents a fixed percentage relative to the tumor SUV_{max}. Most reports use the value of 40–50 %; however with these thresholds, this technique may underestimate the size of the GTV, particularly when the primary tumor is large with inhomogeneous FDG uptake, as is often the case with lymphoma. On the other hand, using lower thresholds may overestimate the tumor volume and include areas that do not represent disease. A recent retrospective analysis of pediatric and young adult patients with HL demonstrated that applying SUV_{max} thresholds from 15 to 40 % led to significant variations on INRT treatment volumes and the optimum starting threshold may be somewhere between 15 and 20 %, with the caveat that this low threshold will often include areas of physiologic uptake that must be carefully excluded by the trained eye with input from a nuclear medicine physician [47].

5.4.4 Other Automated Segmentation Methods

More complex algorithms have been described in the literature for metabolic tumor volume (MTV) assessment, based on a tumor contouring approach, using a predefined cutoff value of the measured activity inside the tumor compared to the surrounding background: the tumor to background (*T/B*) ratio [10]. The advantage of this method is that it is independent of tracer uptake in tumor, which can be quite heterogeneous in HL. The main disadvantage is that it relies on quantifying background uptake, which is fraught with challenges similar to SUV calculation with inherent technical and statistical errors. In order to address the issue with edge detection, numerous publications have reported the successful use of complex algorithms and adaptive thresholding methods [12].

Although there have been many approaches to auto-segmentation described in the literature, each approach has limitations that preclude its implementation as standard of care. Most experts agree that automated or semiautomated methods should be aimed at reducing variability rather than replacing human operation, but we do not know the ideal way to use PET for target volume delineation. Given that the qualitative visual method (with knowledge of quantitative parameters such as SUV) is still the primary method of incorporating PET into RT planning, there is a need for a multidisciplinary assessment of patients upfront before chemotherapy in order to have an accurate assessment of regions involved with disease for the application of smaller radiation treatment fields.

5.4.5 PET Imaging Protocols

Although most information on PET scan results can be gathered with visual assessment in daily practice, the quantitative readings could in theory give some advantages, by providing information on a continuous variable such as the intensity of FDG uptake by the tumor. Quantitative metrics for FDG uptake measurement is critical in response assessment, staging, and RT planning. Imaging protocols are designed to make results reproducible between patients. As such, they are often rigorous and must be consistently applied in order to generate the most meaningful information. Some PET scanners are located within radiation oncology departments and other institutions

rely on PET scans obtained in the nuclear medicine department. Regardless of the location of the PET scanner, the quality control is still important [33, 35]. In 2008, shortly after INRT was introduced in Europe, the International Atomic Energy Agency published guidelines summarizing two consensus meetings regarding the role of PET in radiation treatment planning. These guidelines clearly state that when PET scans are to be used for radiation planning, all of the tools used for patient immobilization should be available including customized molds and face masks. All images should be obtained on a flat tabletop (similar to the radiation treatment table). Furthermore, laser beams should be installed for patient alignment and the gantry aperture must permit a range of patient positions, including arms up and arms akimbo [24]. Of course, this represents the ideal situation. Often, stand-alone pretreatment PET/CT images are all we have available, in which case a great deal of caution must be used when transferring the PET or PET/CT into the RT planning software workstation and the PET imaging should be checked for correct normalization and SUV quantification.

As previously described, RT planning after chemotherapy is based on the pre-chemo extent of disease unless disease progression has occurred. Ideally, the radiation oncologist should see the patient at diagnosis and obtain CT and PET/CT in the treatment position to allow for ease of contouring at the time of treatment. The treatment position in lymphoma varies depending on clinical factors including areas of disease involvement as well as patient age and normal tissue exposure. For the most part, arms will either be raised or akimbo with neck extended in cases that require irradiation of cervical nodes or Waldeyer's ring. This includes imaging with immobilization devices where appropriate. If the radiation oncology facility is not equipped with a PET/CT scanner or if pre-chemo imaging in the treatment position is not available, then co-registration must take place.

Fusing the pretreatment PET/CT directly to the posttreatment, CT has the advantage of providing physiologic data with precise topographic localization and is preferred over side-by-side imaging. Metwally et al. assessed the inter-observer variability in CTV definitions when pre-treatment PET/CTs were either co-registered to posttreatment planning CTs or evaluated with side-by-side imaging. The authors found that registration of the PET/CT and planning CT images resulted in significantly greater consistency of tumor volume definition [34].

5.4.6 Concept of Dose Escalation

In an attempt to better understand the biological significance of FDG-avid areas of tumor in HL, Girinsky et al. measured the degree of shrinkage in the FDG-avid volume of tumor compared to non-FDG-avid volume after treatment with chemotherapy [16]. The hypothesis was that FDG-avid areas of disease may demonstrate less response to chemotherapy and would therefore benefit from receiving higher doses of radiation therapy (also known as dose escalation or dose painting). However, responses after chemotherapy were similar for both FDG-avid and non-FDG-avid lesions (67 and 68 % decrease in size, respectively). In addition, on average 25 % of the volume of disease at baseline was FDG avid (range 0–54 %), suggesting that about 75 % of the tumor mass would not have been visualized if the PET had been performed alone. The authors conclude that dose escalation based on FDG avidity is not a reasonable treatment strategy in HL. Although this study does not support the use of dose escalation based on FDG avidity, there may be other imaging bio-markers that hold promise in determining which patients and which lesions are more likely to recur and would therefore benefit from more aggressive local therapy.

5.5 FDG-PET: Pitfalls and Artifacts Relevant to RT Planning

Although PET has high sensitivity in HL, there can be a number of false positives [31], particularly when interpreted by radiologists or nuclear medicine physicians who lack experience in the pediatric lymphoma population [27]. Multiple noncancerous conditions can mimic lymphoma such as thermogenic brown fat (also known as brown adipose tissue (BAT)), strained muscle, infections, transforming germinal centers in normal lymphatic tissue, thymic hyperplasia, and general inflammatory conditions such as granulomatous diseases (e.g. sarcoidosis) (see Chapter 6).

5.5.1 Organ Motion

One must keep in mind that PET images are acquired over a relatively long period of time (more than 20') and therefore lesions that are subject to motion related to the breathing cycle may appear larger than their actual size. This also has an impact on partial volume effect, where the tumor SUV is underestimated. We do not typically use respiratory gating during PET/CT acquisition but this could be considered moving forward if PET if PET alone were to be used for target volume delineation.

5.5.2 Brown Adipose Tissue

BAT as opposed to white adipose tissue (WAT) is capable of generating heat in response to cold exposure or food ingestion as a consequence of its unique ability to uncouple oxidative phosphorylation in mitochondria. Hence, heat is generated rather than ATP during metabolism. The metabolism of glucose during this process is via the anaerobic pathway and a greater amount of glucose is required in order to provide the ATP for fatty acid oxidation. For this reason BAT is a potential source of false positives in PET scans. Brown fat is more common in children and females, is characteristically not associated with a radiographic or clinical abnormality, and typically has a curvilinear distribution in the neck and supraclavicular areas. This highlights the importance of contouring with FDG-PET co-registered with a CT scan to provide superior anatomic localization of all PET abnormalities. This abnor-

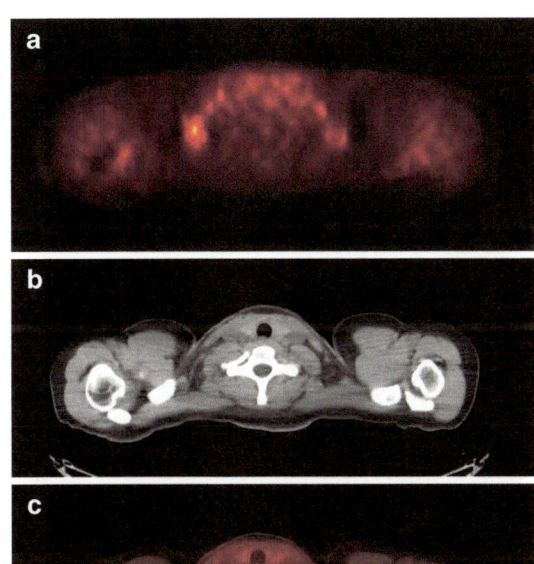

the rate of mild FDG uptake associated with a normal thymus has been estimated to be about 50 % [37]. Some studies have shown that physiologic uptake can be seen in older patients as well [36]. Another cause of thymic uptake is thymic hyperplasia. This phenomenon is associated with chemotherapy, particularly in children with lymphoma, but can also be seen in adults [5]. A critical evaluation of the thymus may be necessary in radiation planning given that it is not uncommon for the thymus to be involved with mediastinal HL, more commonly in the nodular sclerosis subtype [48]. The recognition of physiologic uptake from involvement with HL is particularly important in the era of more conformal radiation techniques. In equivocal cases, other imaging modalities such as MRI can be useful to differentiate benign thymic uptake from malignancy.

Fig. 5.5 FDG uptake due to brown adipose tissue demonstrated on (**a**) PET, (**b**) CT, and (**c**) co-registered PET/CT. Note the absence of tissue density in the region of FDG uptake, a classic finding associated with brown adipose tissue

5.5.4 Physiologic FDG Uptake

We must keep in mind that FDG uptake also occurs in nonmalignant tissue other than brown fat and the thymus [9, 43]. FDG accumulation is actually most notable in the brain and heart due to the presence of glycolytic metabolism. Because FDG is excreted through the urinary system, FDG activity will be present in the kidney's intrarenal collecting system, the ureters, and the bladder. Less intense radiotracer activity is present in the liver, spleen, and bone marrow. Variable physiologic uptake can occur in the digestive tract as well. It is not uncommon for focal uptake to occur at the GE junction. Uptake in the digestive system could easily be assumed to represent subdiaphragmatic lymphadenopathy without correlation to anatomic cross-sectional imaging on CT. In patients who have fasted (which is required for PET scanning), it is not uncommon for the stomach, normal colon, and small intestine to also display FDG uptake. In the bowel, the uptake is typically isolated rather than diffuse and its linear configuration allows the correct identification as uptake limited to the normal bowel. Other areas that can also lead to FDG uptake include the skeletal muscle, thyroid, and bone marrow.

mal uptake is also present in adipose tissue in other parts of the body, specifically in the mediastinum and perinephric fat. The incidence of FDG-avid adipose tissue has been estimated to be between 2 and 6 % depending on the series and can be easily misinterpreted as additional areas of pathologic lymphadenopathy [8]. Measurement of SUV is not always helpful in differentiating between malignant and benign etiology. In one series, the SUV associated with BAT was reported as high as 20 [51]. An example of FDG uptake due to brown adipose tissue is shown in Fig. 5.5.

5.5.3 Thymic FDG Uptake

It is generally accepted that some degree of thymic FDG uptake can be expected until puberty, at which point the thymus undergoes fatty infiltration and involutes. In these prepubescent patients,

5.5.5 Benign Pathologic Causes of FDG Uptake

Benign pathologic FDG uptake can occur in lymph nodes, posing problems in using PET/CT for RT planning in HL. One must be aware that active granulomatous disease such as sarcoidosis and tuberculosis can also cause uptake in lymph nodes [32]. Healing bone and degenerative joints and other sites of infection or inflammation can all cause an increase in FDG that may mimic malignancy [45].

References

1. Aleman BMP, van den Belt-Dusebout AW, Klokman WJ, et al. Long-term cause-specific mortality of patients treated for Hodgkin's disease. J Clin Oncol. 2003;21:3431–9. doi:10.1200/JCO.2003.07.131.

2. Alkhawaldeh K, Alavi A. Quantitative assessment of FDG uptake in brown fat using standardized uptake value and dual-time-point scanning. Clin Nucl Med. 2008;33:663–7.doi:10.1097/RLU.0b013e318184b3de.

3. Bhatia S, Robison LL, Oberlin O, et al. Breast cancer and other second neoplasms after childhood Hodgkin's disease. N Engl J Med. 1996;334:745–51. doi:10.1056/NEJM199603213341201.

4. Boellaard R, Krak NC, Hoekstra OS, Lammertsma AA. Effects of noise, image resolution, and ROI definition on the accuracy of standard uptake values: a simulation study. J Nucl Med. 2004;45:1519–27.

5. Brink I, Reinhardt MJ, Hoegerle S, et al. Increased metabolic activity in the thymus gland studied with 18 F-FDG PET: age dependency and frequency after chemotherapy. J Nucl Med. 2001;42:591–5.

6. Brinker H. A re-analysis of available dose-response and time-dose data in Hodgkin's disease. Radiother Oncol. 1994;30:227.

7. Cheson BD, Pfistner B, Juweid ME, et al. Revised response criteria for malignant lymphoma. J Clin Oncol. 2007;25:579–86. doi:10.1200/JCO.2006.09.2403.

8. Cohade C, Osman M, Pannu HK, Wahl RL. Uptake in supraclavicular area fat ("USA-fat"): description on 18F-FDG PET/CT. J Nucl Med. 2003;44:170–6.

9. Cook GJR, Fogelman I, Maisey MN. Normal physiological and benign pathological variants of 18-fluoro-2-deoxyglucose positron-emission tomography scanning: potential for error in interpretation. Semin Nucl Med. 1996;26:308–14. doi:10.1016/S0001-2998(96)80006-7.

10. Daisne J-F, Sibomana M, Bol A, et al. Tri-dimensional automatic segmentation of PET volumes based on measured source-to-background ratios: influence of reconstruction algorithms. Radiother Oncol. 2003;69:247–50. doi:10.1016/S0167-8140(03)00270-6.

11. Devita VT. Combination chemotherapy in the treatment of advanced Hodgkin's disease. Ann Intern Med. 1970;73:881. doi:10.7326/0003-4819-73-6-881.

12. Drever L, Wilson R, McEwan A, et al. Comparison of three image segmentation techniques for target volume delineation in positron emission tomography. J Appl Clin Med Phys. 2007;8:93–109.

13. Freudenberg LS, Antoch G, Schütt P, et al. FDG-PET/CT in re-staging of patients with lymphoma. Eur J Nucl Med Mol Imaging. 2004;31:325–9. doi:10.1007/s00259-003-1375-y.

14. Geworski L, Knoop BO, de Wit M, et al. Multicenter comparison of calibration and cross calibration of PET scanners. J Nucl Med. 2002;43:635–9.

15. Gilbert R. Radiotherapy in Hodgkin's disease (malignant granulomatosis). Am J Roentgenol. 1939;41:198–241.

16. Girinsky T, Ghalibafian M, Bonniaud G, et al. Is FDG-PET scan in patients with early stage Hodgkin lymphoma of any value in the implementation of the involved-node radiotherapy concept and dose painting? Radiother Oncol. 2007;85:178–86. doi:10.1016/j.radonc.2007.07.003.

17. Girinsky T, Specht L, Ghalibafian M, et al. The conundrum of Hodgkin lymphoma nodes: to be or not to be included in the involved node radiation fields. The EORTC-GELA lymphoma group guidelines. Radiother Oncol. 2008;88:202–10. doi:10.1016/j.radonc.2008.05.012.

18. Girinsky T, van der Maazen R, Specht L, et al. Involved-node radiotherapy (INRT) in patients with early Hodgkin lymphoma: concepts and guidelines. Radiother Oncol. 2006;79:270–7. doi:10.1016/j.radonc.2006.05.015.

19. Graham M, Peterson L, Hayward R. Comparison of simplified quantitative analyses of FDG uptake. Nucl Med Biol. 2000;27:647–55. doi:10.1016/S0969-8051(00)00143-8.

20. Gregoire V. Is there any future in radiotherapy planning without the use of PET: unraveling the myth…. Radiother Oncol. 2004;73:261–3. doi:10.1016/j.radonc.2004.10.005.

21. Hancock SL, Hoppe RT, Horning SJ, Rosenberg SA. Intercurrent death after Hodgkin disease therapy in radiotherapy and adjuvant MOPP trials. Ann Intern Med. 1988;109:183–9.

22. Hong R, Halama J, Bova D, et al. Correlation of PET standard uptake value and CT window-level thresholds for target delineation in CT-based radiation treatment planning. Int J Radiat Oncol Biol Phys. 2007;67:720–6. doi:10.1016/j.ijrobp.2006.09.039.

23. Hutchings M, Loft A, Hansen M, et al. Clinical impact of FDG-PET/CT in the planning of radiotherapy for early-stage Hodgkin lymphoma. Eur J Haematol. 2007;78:206–12. doi:10.1111/j.1600-0609.2006.00802.x.

24. International Atomic Energy Agency (IAEA). IAEA-TECDOC-1603: the role of PET/CT in radiation treatment planning for cancer patient treatment. 2008.

25. Kaplan HS. The radical radiotherapy of regionally localized Hodgkin's disease. Radiology. 1962;78:553–61. doi:10.1148/78.4.553.

26. Kaplan S. The treatment of Hodgkin's disease. Med Clin North Am. 1966;50:1591–610.

27. Kaste SC, Howard SC, McCarville EB, et al. 18 F-FDG-avid sites mimicking active disease in pediatric Hodgkin's. Pediatr Radiol. 2005;35:141–54. doi:10.1007/s00247-004-1340-3.

28. Kim CK, Gupta NC. Dependency of standardized uptake values of fluorine-18 fluorodeoxyglucose on body size: comparison of body surface area correction and lean body mass correction. Nucl Med Commun. 1996;17:890–4.

29. Krasin MJ, Hudson MM, Kaste SC. Positron emission tomography in pediatric radiation oncology: integration in the treatment-planning process. Pediatr Radiol. 2004;34:214–21. doi:10.1007/s00247-003-1113-4.

30. Lee YK, Cook G, Flower MA, et al. Addition of 18F-FDG-PET scans to radiotherapy planning of thoracic lymphoma. Radiother Oncol. 2004;73:277–83. doi:10.1016/j.radonc.2004.07.029.

31. Levine JM, Weiner M, Kelly KM. Routine use of PET scans after completion of therapy in pediatric Hodgkin disease results in a high false positive rate. J Pediatr Hematol Oncol. 2006;28:711–4. doi:10.1097/01.mph.0000243648.66734.eb.

32. Lewis PJ, Salama A. Uptake of fluorine-18-fluorodeoxyglucose in sarcoidosis. J Nucl Med. 1994;35:1647–9.

33. Lucignani G, Jereczek-Fossa BA, Orecchia R. The role of molecular imaging in precision radiation therapy for target definition, treatment planning optimisation and quality control. Eur J Nucl Med Mol Imaging. 2004;31:1059–63. doi:10.1007/s00259-004-1517-x.

34. Metwally H, Courbon F, David I, et al. Coregistration of prechemotherapy PET-CT for planning pediatric Hodgkin's disease radiotherapy significantly diminishes interobserver variability of clinical target volume definition. Int J Radiat Oncol Biol Phys. 2011;80:793–9. doi:10.1016/j.ijrobp.2010.02.024.

35. Mutic S, Dempsey JF, Bosch WR, et al. Multimodality image registration quality assurance for conformal three-dimensional treatment planning. Int J Radiat Oncol. 2001;51:255–60. doi:10.1016/S0360-3016(01)01659-5.

36. Nakahara T, Fujii H, Ide M, et al. FDG uptake in the morphologically normal thymus: comparison of FDG positron emission tomography and CT. Br J Radiol. 2001;74:821–4. doi:10.1259/bjr.74.885.740821.

37. Patel PM, Alibazoglu H, Ali A, et al. Normal thymic uptake of FDG on PET imaging. Clin Nucl Med. 1996;21:772–5.

38. Paulino AC, Margolin J, Dreyer Z, et al. Impact of PET-CT on involved field radiotherapy design for pediatric Hodgkin lymphoma. Pediatr Blood Cancer. 2012;58(6):860–4. doi:10.1002/pbc.23273.

39. Peters M. A study of survivals in Hodgkin's disease treated radiologically. Am J Roentgenol Radium Ther. 1950;63:299–311.

40. Pusey WA. Cases of sarcoma and of Hodgkin's disease treated by exposures to x-rays—a preliminary report. JAMA J Am Med Assoc. 1902;XXXVIII:166. doi:10.1001/jama.1902.62480030024001h.

41. Robertson VL, Anderson CS, Keller FG, et al. Role of FDG-PET in the definition of involved-field radiation therapy and management for pediatric Hodgkin's lymphoma. Int J Radiat Oncol Biol Phys. 2011;80:324–32. doi:10.1016/j.ijrobp.2010.02.002.

42. Shahidi M, Kamangari N, Ashley S, et al. Site of relapse after chemotherapy alone for stage I and II Hodgkin's disease. Radiother Oncol. 2006;78:1–5. doi:10.1016/j.radonc.2005.10.018.

43. Shreve PD, Anzai Y, Wahl RL. Pitfalls in oncologic diagnosis with FDG PET imaging: physiologic and benign variants. Radiographics. 1999;19:61–77. doi:10.1148/radiographics.19.1.g99ja0761, quiz 150–1.

44. Specht L, Yahalom J, Illidge T, et al. Modern radiation therapy for Hodgkin lymphoma: field and dose guidelines from the international lymphoma radiation oncology group (ILROG). Int J Radiat Oncol Biol Phys. 2014;89:854–62. doi:10.1016/j.ijrobp.2013.05.005.

45. Strauss LG. Fluorine-18 deoxyglucose and false-positive results: a major problem in the diagnostics of oncological patients. Eur J Nucl Med. 1996;23:1409–15.

46. Terezakis SA, Hunt MA, Kowalski A, et al. [18F] FDG-positron emission tomography coregistration with computed tomography scans for radiation treatment planning of lymphoma and hematologic malignancies. Int J Radiat Oncol Biol Phys. 2011;81:615–22. doi:10.1016/j.ijrobp.2010.06.044.

47. Walker AJ, Chirindel A, Hobbs RF, et al. Use of standardized uptake value thresholding for target volume delineation in pediatric Hodgkin lymphoma. Pract Radiat Oncol. 2015;5:219–27. doi:10.1016/j.prro.2014.12.004.

48. Wernecke K, Vassallo P, Rutsch F, et al. Thymic involvement in Hodgkin disease: CT and sonographic findings. Radiology. 1991;181:375–83. doi:10.1148/radiology.181.2.1924775.

49. Yahalom J, Mauch P. The involved field is back: issues in delineating the radiation field in Hodgkin's disease. Ann Oncol. 2002;13 Suppl 1:79–83. doi:10.1093/annonc/mdf616.

50. Yaremko B, Riauka T, Robinson D, et al. Thresholding in PET images of static and moving targets. Phys Med Biol. 2005;50:5969–82. doi:10.1088/0031-9155/50/24/014.

51. Yeung HWD, Grewal RK, Gonen M, et al. Patterns of (18)F-FDG uptake in adipose tissue and muscle: a potential source of false-positives for PET. J Nucl Med. 2003;44:1789–96.

Alberto Biggi

Abbreviations

5-PS	Five-Point Scale
AIMN	Associazione Italiana di Medicina Nucleare
BM	Bone Marrow
CT	Computed Tomography
DLBCL	Diffuse Large B-Cell Lymphoma
EANM	European Association of Nuclear Medicine
FDG	^{18}F-Fluoro-Deoxyglucose
HL	Hodgkin Lymphoma
HRS	Hodgkin and Reed-Sternberg Cells
PET	Positron Emission Tomography
SNM	Society of Nuclear Medicine
SUV	Standardized Uptake Value

6.1 Introduction

The medical report is "a written document by which the specialist states conform to the truth the results of diagnostic imaging, together with the clinical interpretation of the results themselves, in relation to the clinical and medical history" [1].

A. Biggi, MD
Nuclear Medicine Department, ASO Santa Croce e
Carle, Cuneo, Italy
e-mail: biggi.a@ospedale.cuneo.it

The medical report is a structured as a formal vehicle for a written and understandable communication between the doctors and eventually between the doctors and the legal system. It represents the subjective interpretation of physical findings in images by the specialist (either nuclear medicine physician or radiologist), is based on the semiotics of a given imaging technique, and provides the answer to the clinical questions arisen by the treating physician. The content of each report will vary according to the exact circumstances concerning each case. While a degree of flexibility is necessary to encompass all the relevant points, a structured framework for the reporting document is strongly recommended. In general, the PET/CT report (a) describes the presence or absence of abnormal FDG accumulation in the PET images in combination with their size and intensity, (b) correlates these findings to other diagnostic tests and interprets them in that context, and (c) contextualizes imaging findings in the available clinical information in order to reply to specific question posed by the clinician.

The aim of this chapter is to suggest a minimum of dataset for PET reporting in lymphoma according to previously published guidelines or recommendations by EANM [2], SNM [3], AIMN [4], the expert session "How to report a baseline and end of treatment PET scan" held in Menton (France), September 18th, 2014 [5], the "Consensus of the International Conference on Malignant Lymphomas Imaging Working Group"

© Springer International Publishing Switzerland 2016
A. Gallamini (ed.), *PET Scan in Hodgkin Lymphoma*, DOI 10.1007/978-3-319-31797-7_6

[6, 7], and the author's personal experience. Finally, the framework for PET/CT reporting in lymphoma presented in this chapter has been drawn in accord with the general semiotics elements of nuclear medicine for clinical reporting.

6.2 Image Requirements for Reporting

Reporting is performed on reconstructed PET and CT images displayed on workstation screen. The software packages for current PET/CT systems enable visualization of PET, CT, and PET + CT fusion images in the axial, coronal, and sagittal planes as well as intensity projections in a 3D cine mode. PET images can be displayed with and without attenuation correction. On the attenuation-corrected images, quantitative information with respect to size and FDG uptake can be derived. Images must be evaluated using software and monitors approved for clinical use in nuclear medicine. Both uncorrected and attenuation-corrected images need to be assessed in order to identify any artifact caused by contrasts agent, metal implants, and/or patient motion. PET scans are best reported using a fixed display and color table scaled to the SUV to assist with consistency of reporting, for serial scans, and to reduce the effect of patient size.

6.3 How to Interpret PET/CT Images at Baseline and After Treatment

PET/CT has been used long since for pretreatment tumor burden assessment and staging purposes, as well as for treatment response assessment [8]. Tumor stage is just one of the prognostic indices increasingly used for pretreatment risk stratification and therapy selection. Recently a modification of the Ann Arbor classification for anatomic description of disease extension was proposed [7]. PET/CT is generally assessed using visual criteria; the SUV is cur-

rently used as a semiquantitative measure of the degree of FDG uptake, but it is not a determinant tool for scan interpretation. The detection limits of PET depend on the degree of contrast between the tumor and its immediate surroundings. PET is an intrinsically quantitative imaging technique and there are in principle no definite limits to the intensity of FDG uptake by the tissues. The latter, in turn, depends on histology (FDG avidity of the type of lymphoma), the burden of viable tumor cells, movement during acquisition (e.g., blurred signals in the case of pulmonary, hepatic, or splenic foci), and physiological uptake in the adjacent background. Although variable and depending on the clinical context, it has been demonstrated that the detection power of FDG-PET declines with the reduction of tumor diameter, being very low or absent for tumors with a diameter $\leq$6–8 mm, even in very FDG-avid tumors. The main criteria to report a PET/CT for staging purpose in lymphoma have been recently reviewed [9]. The typical finding of an abnormal scan is usually defined by a pathological focal FDG uptake in nodal and extranodal sites, including the spleen, liver, marrow/bone, or other organs. FDG accumulation should be visually compared to the background uptake in, e.g., mediastinum blood pool (MBPS) and the liver and reported as mild ($\leq$ MBPS), moderate (> MBPS $\leq$ liver), or intense (> liver).

The hallmark of spleen involvement by lymphoma consists in a single or multiple areas of focal uptake with an activity higher than the liver with/without an enlarged spleen (longitudinal diameter > 13 cm) [10]. Both focal and diffuse uptakes with an activity higher than the liver are considered an harbinger of disease in non-Hodgkin lymphoma (NHL), while in Hodgkin lymphoma (HL), a histologic proof of organ involvement by disease has been reported only in presence a focal FDG uptake [10]. By converse, a diffuse uptake is frequently associated in HL with a diffuse bone marrow (BM) uptake and is more likely to represent inflammation due to chemokines produced by the Hodgkin and Reed-Sternberg cells (HRS) and no evidence of spleen invasion by lymphoma. On the other hand, the association of splenomegaly and diffuse splenic uptake, with an intensity higher than the normal liver, may be suspicious of splenic involvement. There is not a given, definite pattern of FDG uptake which is deemed to portrait bone/bone marrow involvement (BMI) by lymphoma. While in HL and DLBCL in most cases, BMI is typically displayed by a focal FDG uptake with an intensity higher than the liver, in some cases diffuse uptake has been described in DLBCL [11–13]. By contrast, in follicular lymphoma (FL) bone marrow involvement is typically diffuse [14, 15]. Using PET/CT it is not possible and not strictly indispensable to distinguish with certainty BM from bone involvement, because in both cases the stage of the disease is the same. Moreover, the limits of space resolution and detection power of the currently available scanner equipment often preclude the distinction between cortical or spongy bone invasion by lymphoma. However, in general, the presence of areas of focal FDG uptake associated with abnormalities on CT, seen as osteolytic, sclerotic, or mixed lesions, support bone infiltration involvement, while the absence of abnormalities on CT supports BM infiltration only. Focal FDG uptake associated with abnormalities on CT may be also related to benign non-lymphomatous process including osteoporotic changes of vertebral body, spondylosis, osteoarthritis, fractures, osteomyelitis, osteoid osteoma, etc., often yielding false-positive results in PET and fused PET/CT images. Considering the CT criteria of these lesions will largely eliminate false-positive results regardless their uptake value. Thus, in combined PET/CT, CT images significantly improve PET specificity with better localization of bone involvement in case of focal BMI. On the other hand, PET can detect BM-based localization early and in the absence of morphologic changes on CT images, both in cases of focal and diffuse BMI by lymphoma, thereby improving CT sensitivity. The influence of the integration of PET and CT upon CT specificity is also notable in cases of treated healed bony lesions, which lack metabolic activity in spite of a suspicious morphologic appearance. In general an abnormal accumulation persisting longer than 3 months in a fracture site is likely due to either osteomyelitis or malignancy. A diffuse homogeneous uptake in BM is frequently associated with a diffuse increase of splenic uptake in HL and is more likely to represent inflammation due to chemokines. In NHL a diffusely increased BM uptake that is greater than that of the normal liver should be considered compatible with lymphoma unless the patient history discloses a recent cytokine administration. Lymphoma spread in other extranodal sites usually presents as a focal area of uptake with an activity usually higher than the liver uptake and is associated with an abnormal finding on the CT part of the PET/CT.

PET/CT is generally assessed using visual criteria after treatment also, and the 5-PS is recommended for reporting [6, 7]. Meanwhile, it is suggested, according to published data, that score 4 be applied to uptake > the maximum SUV in a large region of normal liver and score 5 to uptake 2X to 3X the maximum SUV in the liver. The 5-PS (so called Deauville score) criteria follow the continuum of uptake with the likelihood of malignancy increasing with the level of FDG uptake and were intended to be an objective reporting method, easy to understand, and to implement in different centers that would be reproducible when used by reporters in different countries. The 5-PS allow the outcome in patients with different levels of residual uptake to be analyzed; a high negative predictive value is desirable when de-escalation of therapy is proposed in patients with a good prognosis, while a high positive predictive value is desirable when intensification of therapy is proposed in patients with a poor prognosis. According to the 5-PS, the score of the patients is related to the activity of the most active lesion in the patient, i.e., to the activity of the "reference lesion" that is identified by scaling and eventually measuring its activity (SUVMax). A more detailed set of instructions was drawn up to deal with potential confounding variables in the interpretation of the interim and final PET [16].

6.4 What Is Normal and Abnormal in PET Images at Baseline and After Treatment?

The typical finding of an abnormal scan in lymphoma is usually defined by a focal pathological FDG uptake in nodal and extranodal sites. However soon after the introduction of FDG-PET for human studies, it became clear that FDG-PET imaging is not specific for cancer because nonphysiological variable uptake of FDG occurs in many tissues and in lesions characterized by a substantial presence of inflammatory cells. Therefore, as it is possible that benign and malignant lesions are present simultaneously in a single patient, it is not possible to know with certainty in a given imaging technique (either PET or CT) the pathology counterpart of the identified lesion. Accordingly, as taking a biopsy of all the sites of disease turns out unfeasible and unethical, it is difficult to clearly define what should be considered the "gold standard" reference for a given imaging technique for assessing its overall accuracy. In clinical practice, the need of a biopsy should be limited to those cases in which this information can change the stage of disease, at diagnosis, or the therapeutic choice during or at the end of treatment. A proper interpretation and accurate characterization of an abnormality detected in PET/CT could be given by complying with a narrow definition of "lesion" (area of focal uptake of tracer which corresponds to a CT imaging abnormalities, which is not explained by other causes than tumor) in the awareness of the conditions and the mechanisms yielding false-positive and false-negative results. Many articles in the current literature report about physiological and nonphysiological FDG accumulations observed in PET/CT and about pitfalls or artifacts observed at baseline and after treatment [17–20]. A physiological and variable FDG accumulation can be observed to a certain degree in most viable tissue like the brain, myocardium, breast, liver, spleen, stomach, intes-

tine, kidneys, urine, skeletal muscle, lymphatic tissue, bone marrow, salivary glands, thymus, uterus, ovaries, and testicles. In whole-body PET/CT examinations, the brain shows a high FDG accumulation. For the detection of brain localization, FDG-PET is therefore only of limited value and thus FDG-PET is usually not used for the primary detection or exclusion of brain metastases.

A nonphysiological, variable and nonspecific FDG accumulation can be observed in brown fat, in myocardium, in granulation tissue (e.g., wound healing), in granulomatous disease (e.g., sarcoidosis), in infections and other inflammatory processes (pneumonia, esophagitis, gastritis, cholangitis, etc.), and in benign non-neoplastic disease (thyroid functioning nodules, adrenal nodules, salivary gland tumors, etc.). The distribution of brown fat includes the neck, axilla, upper mediastinum, and paravertebral region. Variable patterns of intestinal FDG uptake are present in the patients receiving anti-hyperglycemic drugs including metformin, with particularly diffuse, multifocal, or nodular variations with predominance in the large intestine, a lesser presence in the small intestine. The transient discontinuation of metformin therapy for 2 days just before a FDG-PET/CT scan markedly reduces the increased intestinal FDG uptake without causing a significant increase in the blood glucose level [21, 22]. Bone marrow is often suppressed during chemotherapy. To overcome chemotherapy-induced neutropenia, granulocytic colony-stimulating growth factors (G-CSF) are often administered to promote BM repopulation after treatment. Growth factors (G-CSF) rapidly increase BM FDG uptake, but the effects on FDG uptake do not last for more than 2 weeks after the final administration; during and after G-CSF treatment, a sustained increased FDG uptake is also often observed in the spleen, although less frequent and marked as that observed in the bone marrow. Elevated FDG avidity in the BM may also be seen in anemic patients. These findings must be distinguished from malignancy [23, 24]. Thymic hyperplasia after chemotherapy is a common finding among children and adolescents and may also be seen in adults; thymic hyperplasia is allegedly accounted by an immunologic rebound phenomenon that is characterized by lymph follicles with large nuclear centers and infiltration of plasma cells after thymic aplasia. Although this phenomenon usually appears within 2–6 months after completion of chemotherapy and may persist for 12–24 months, in some cases a thymic rebound can develop as early as 1 week after therapy end [25, 26]. Bleomycin is an antibiotic agent with antitumor activity, commonly used as part of the cytostatic treatment in HL. Because of the lack of the bleomycin-inactivating enzyme, bleomycin hydrolase, in the lungs and the skin, bleomycin-induced toxic effect occurs predominantly in these organs. The central event in the development of bleomycin-induced pneumonitis is endothelial damage of the lung vasculature caused by bleomycin-induced cytokines and free radicals. This inflammatory process can result in an increase in pulmonary FDG uptake that may be seen within 2 months after the start of bleomycin treatment [27, 28]. Surgery is a form of tissue injury, and, as expected, it elicits an inflammatory response that can be visualized as an area of increased FDG activity. Postsurgical inflammation will be evident on FDG-PET/CT as FDG-avid soft tissue in the surgical bed; these changes usually resolve in a few weeks. The intensity of tracer uptake depends on the extent of surgery and how the wound was healed: for example, there are few visible signs on PET 10 days after mediastinoscopy but the inflammatory consequences of a sternotomy will remain visible for months. In patients who have undergone radiation therapy, normal tissues close to the boundaries of radiation fields are also, at least in part, exposed, and injury to these tissues often results in FDG-avid inflammation. As the effects of radiotherapy are somewhat longer lasting, end-of-treatment PET scan should be planned not earlier than 8–12

weeks after the end of treatment in order to reduce the post-radiation unspecific FDG uptake. This time frame fits well the clinical context of these patients, rarely experiencing a treatment failure within 3 months after the end of radiation treatment. Radiation pneumonitis is an inflammatory reaction within irradiated lung tissue in response to radiation injury and is characterized by the migration of leukocytes from the blood to irradiated lung tissue; radiation pneumonitis may appear as early as 2 weeks after irradiation and may persist for many months. On FDG-PET scans, radiation pneumonitis will result in elevated FDG avidity. The linear distribution of abnormalities seen on both CT and FDG-PET scans helps distinguish radiation pneumonitis from pulmonary infection or malignancy [29–31]. The interpretation of a FDG uptake by bone in a site previously involved by disease after treatment might be difficult because this phenomenon, especially in presence of a lytic lesions, may be related both to bone healing, which transiently increases FDG uptake, and to a residual disease. In general, in patients with residual disease, the degree of uptake is higher. These clinical observations suggest that an interval of at least 6 weeks should be allowed to minimize the risk of false-positive findings after treatment of bone lesions and of at least 3–6 months should elapse between surgery or traumatic bone lesions and PET scan.

6.5 Other Factors Interfering with PET Interpretation

There are no conclusive data on the optimum interval between chemotherapy and PET. The minimum interval between the last dose of chemotherapy and PET should be 10 days, and the latter should be planned as close as possible to the next treatment administration. This is because of any possible effects on tumor metabolism (such as macrophage impairment) and systemic effect (such as bone marrow activation following bone marrow depression, which may or may not be caused by growth factor).

6.6   How to Write the Clinical Report

PET and CT findings should be integrated in a combined report rather than being reported separately. Typical report includes patient details/demographics, procedure description and imaging protocol, clinical information, clinical report interpretation/conclusion, and author/s.

1. *Patient details/demographics*

Mandatory These data may be country specific but in general they include name and family name, place and birthday of the patient, patient and study identifier, and date of examination.

2. *Procedure description and imaging protocol*

Mandatory The radiopharmaceutical administered and its activity (in MBq), the level of blood glucose before the examination and the diabetic status, the field of view and patient positioning (whole body, skull base, to mid-thigh), the CT protocol (low dose for attenuation correction and image fusion vs full-dose contrast-enhanced CT; the contrast agent should be specified), the actual interval between FDG administration, and the start of acquisition if outside the standard operating procedure (SOP) (SOP: 60 ± 10).

Recorded but not included in the report: Height and weight of the patients, site of injection, extravasation, quality control parameters of the radiopharmaceutical preparation, drug administration (benzodiazepines, beta-blockers, insulin, etc.); method of image reconstruction if outside the SOP (SOP: iterative reconstruction); motion or respiratory artifacts; camera details and quality control parameters; and CT dose.

3. *Clinical indication*

Mandatory Indications for PET/CT examination, i.e., staging, early or interim restaging, and end of therapy restaging.

Recommended Relevant patient history.

4. *Description of findings in PET/CT and CT*

This is the main body of the report; it sets out the information you found when you read PET/CT. The meaning of this information may change in the different type of lymphoma and different time points of patient scanning before, during, and after treatment.

Mandatory *Description of relevant findings likely related to the disease*: PET/CT scans report (1) the anatomical location, the extent, and the intensity of pathological FDG accumulation in nodal and extranodal sites and (2) the relevant morphologic findings related to PET abnormalities on the CT images. The intensity of uptake in the different nodal area and in extranodal sites may be described as mild, moderate, or intense; a quantitative estimate of the intensity of FGD uptake (SUVMax) in the different nodal area can be provided especially if the pattern of uptake is suggestive of transformation (e.g., in follicular lymphoma and in chronic lymphocytic leukemia). Extranodal disease spread should be recorded according to the involved site (the lung, liver, bone/bone marrow, etc.). The dimension of the spleen should be given by measuring its largest diameter on CT scan (splenomegaly if >13 cm). The anatomical location, the activity (SUVMax), and the size of the most active lesion (reference metabolic lesion) and the dimension and location of the largest mass (transverse slice), even if the latter is not the reference metabolic lesion, where feasible, should be provided.

Description of incidental findings in PET/CT which are FDG-avid but unlikely disease-

related, such as focal colonic uptake, diffuse or nodular tracer uptake in thyroid, adrenal adenoma, salivary gland tumors, hilar and mediastinal node in sarcoidosis, etc.. These findings should be described both before and after treatment, with a warning on their nature not attributable to lymphoma (in posttreatment settings they may provide false-positive results).

Description of findings in CT that are relevant to patients care, even in the case they are PET negative. Comment on any potential life threatening or clinically critical finding, e.g., potential spinal cord compression, perforation, superior vena cava obstruction, pleural and pericardial effusion, aortic aneurysm, etc., should be added.

Recommended *Description of the incidental findings in CT* such as renal atrophy, gallstones, etc.

5. *Interpretation/conclusions*

The final interpretation of the findings is hereby reported and the conclusion should be sound to the clinical context in which a PET scan is required.

Mandatory at staging A synthetic comment on area/s of abnormal uptake in nodal and extranodal sites should be included. Whenever feasible, the most probable diagnosis should be given, resulting from a synthesis of the available clinical data and of the semiotics of the abnormal PET findings. When appropriate, a differential diagnosis should be given with an estimated probability of a diagnosis. The location, activity (SUVMax), and dimension of the most active lesion (reference metabolic lesion), the location and dimension of the largest lesion, and the extension of the disease (Ann Arbor or modified Ann Arbor Stage) should be reported. When appropriate, follow-up and additional diagnostic studies to confirm the clinical hypothesis should be recommended, e.g., site for biopsy or lymphoma with suspected transformation.

Report findings in CT that are relevant to patients' care.

Mandatory during and after therapy A synthetic comment on area/s of abnormal uptake, in nodal and extranodal sites, suspect to harbinger residual disease should be included. The location, activity (SUVMax), and dimension of the single most active lesion (reference metabolic lesion) and the location and dimension of the largest lesion should be reported.

The area/s of any new site/s of disease (due to lymphoma or nonspecific) should also be described. All the above information should be displayed by comparing the recorded persisting abnormality with that in the previous PET/CT scan and/or other previous imaging studies and clinical data that are relevant. Finally the Deauville score should be reported using the 5-point Deauville scale. According to the Lugano criteria for lymphoma response assessment, the abnormal (if any) finding recorded in the PET scan should be categorized in one of the following levels: complete metabolic response/partial metabolic response/ stable metabolic disease/progressive metabolic disease. Recommendations for further imaging or investigation if relevant as well as a mention on CT findings that could be relevant for patient care should also be added. Representative case and an example of template for recording sites of involvement are reported in Figs. 6.1, 6.2, 6.3, 6.4, 6.5, 6.6, 6.7, 6.8, 6.9, 6.10, and 6.11

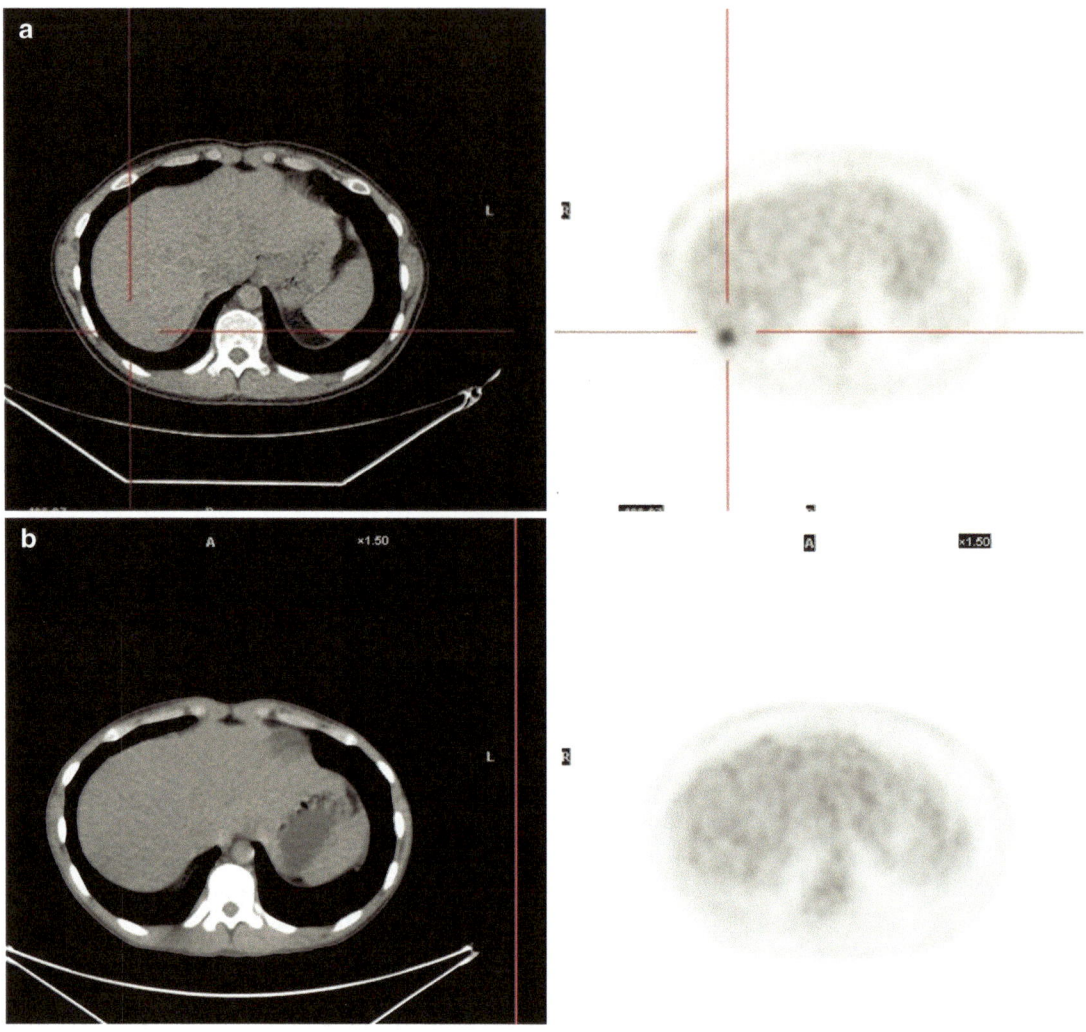

Fig. 6.1 Stage IV HL. Focal uptake in the liver at baseline (**a**) that disappears after treatment (**b**)

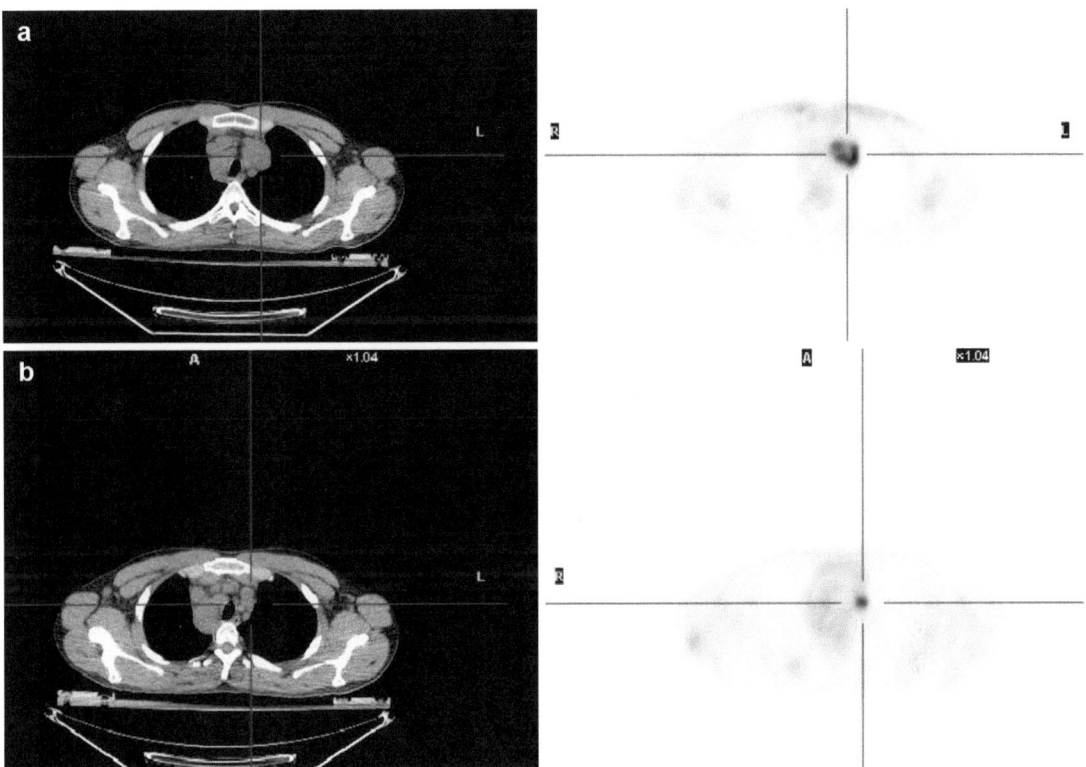

Fig. 6.2   Focal uptake in paratracheal left node at baseline (**a**) and after treatment (score 4) (**b**) in HL

interim PET

baseline PET

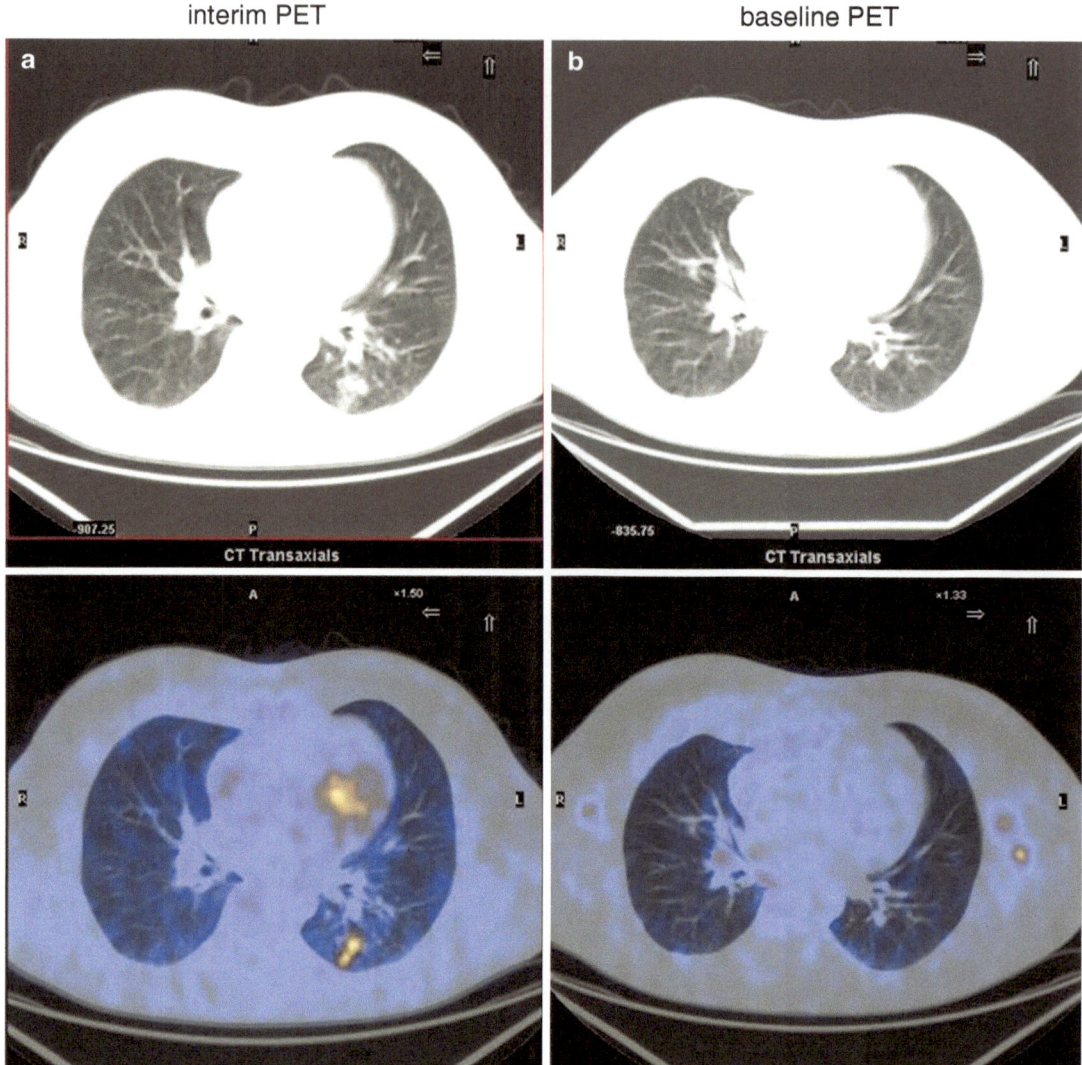

Fig. 6.3 Focal uptake in lung abnormalities in interim PET (**a**) after 2 ABVD not present in baseline PET due to pneumonia; nodes in left axilla present in baseline PET (**b**) were no more evident after treatment

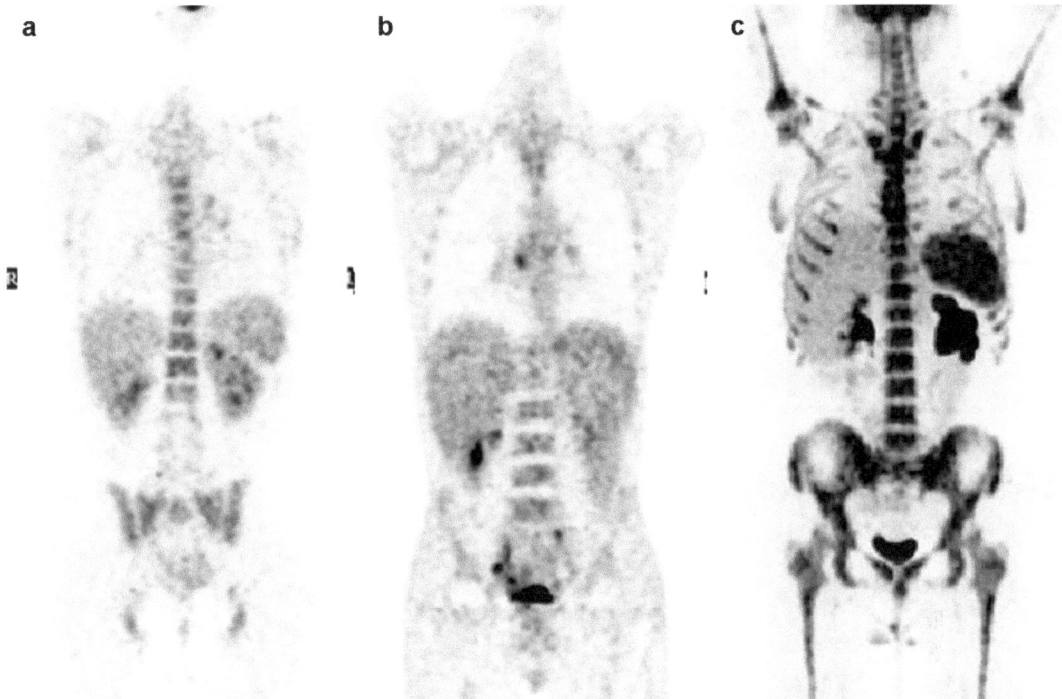

Fig. 6.4 Diffuse uptake in the bone marrow and spleen at baseline PET due to chemokines stimulation produced by the HRS cells in patients with HL (Case **a** and **b**); intense bone marrow and spleen uptake after 3 days of G-CSF treatment 8 days after the last BEACOPP treatment (Case **c**)

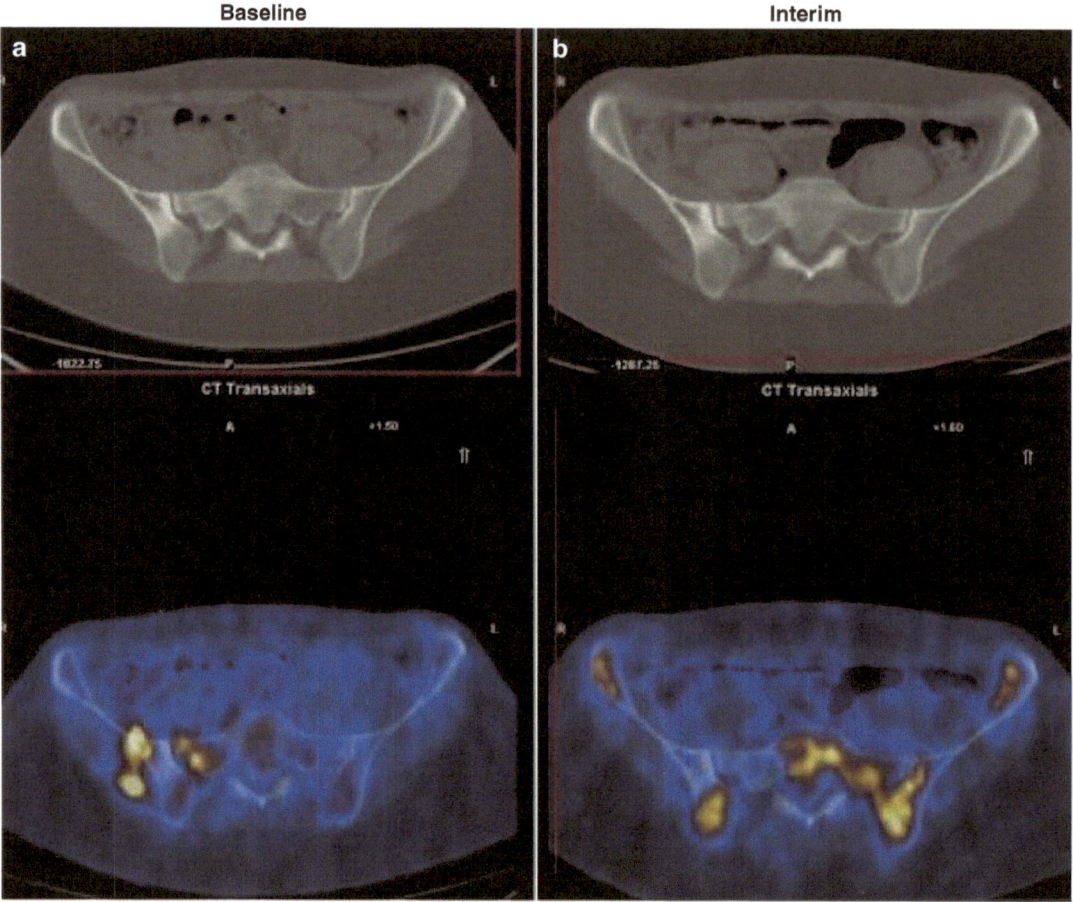

Fig. 6.5 Focal uptake in the right ileum, right sacrum and in the left side of L3 in baseline PET (**a**). After treatment with 2 ABVD (**b**), is evident an increased uptake in normal bone marrow due to chemotherapy effect associated with focal cold areas in bone site previously involved by disease

Baseline   **Interim**

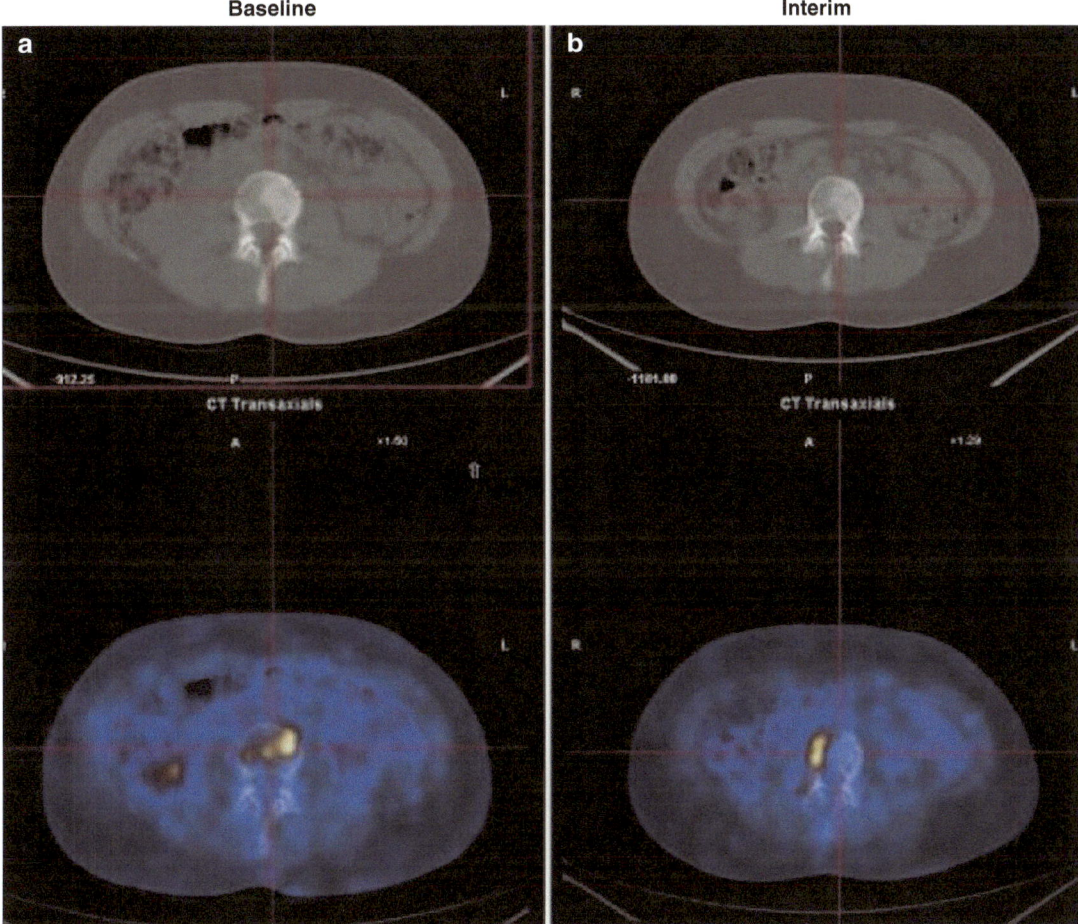

Fig.6.5 (continued)

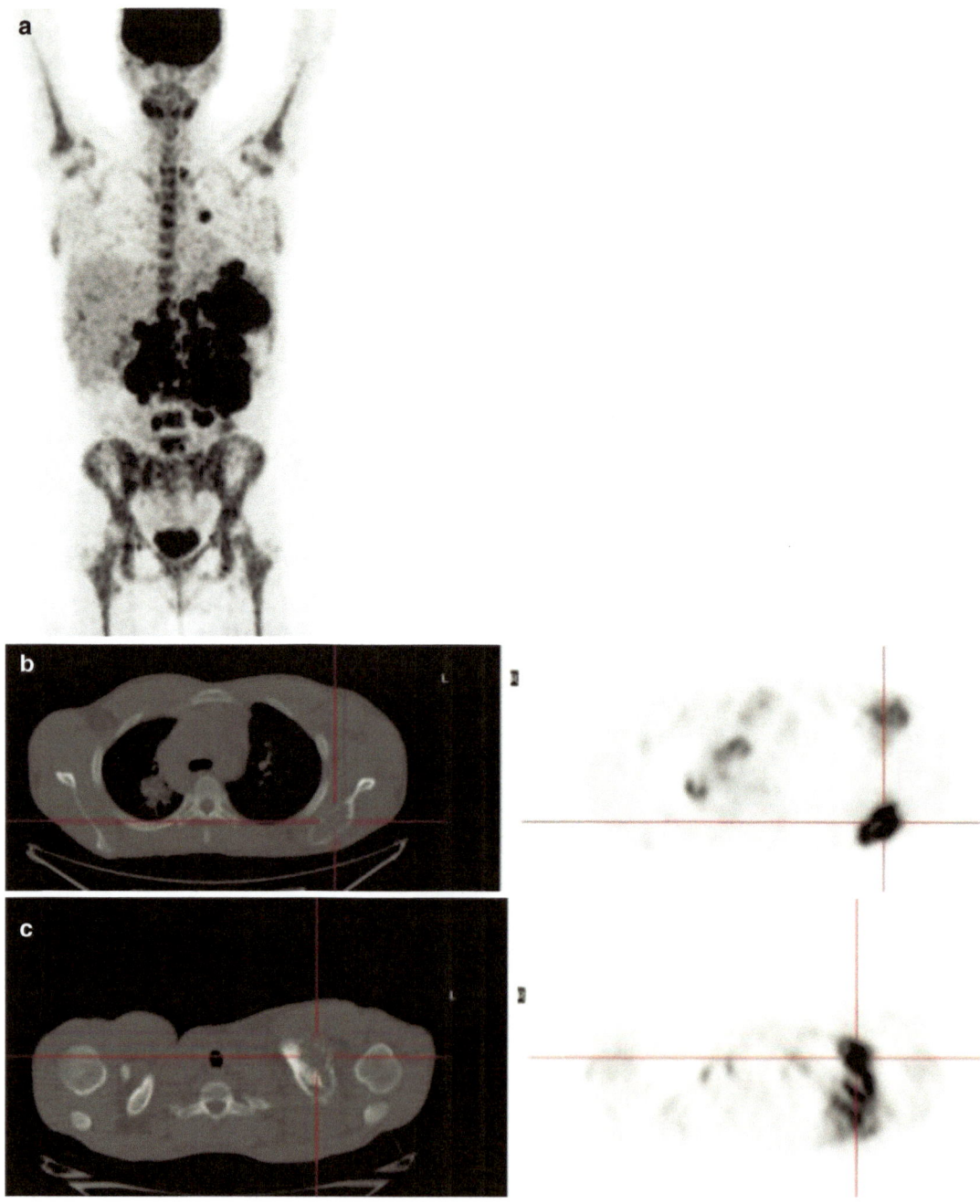

Fig. 6.6 (**a**) Stage IV HL; diffuse bone marrow and spleen uptake due to chemokine stimulation (**a**) associated with lytic lesion in the left scapula (**b**) and in the left clavicula (**c**). (**b**) Interim PET after 2 ABVD; diffuse bone marrow and spleen uptake due to chemotherapy (**d**); diffuse residual uptake in the left scapula due to the healing process of the osteolytic lesion (score 3) (**e**) and focal uptake in the left clavicle due to residual disease (score 4) (**f**)

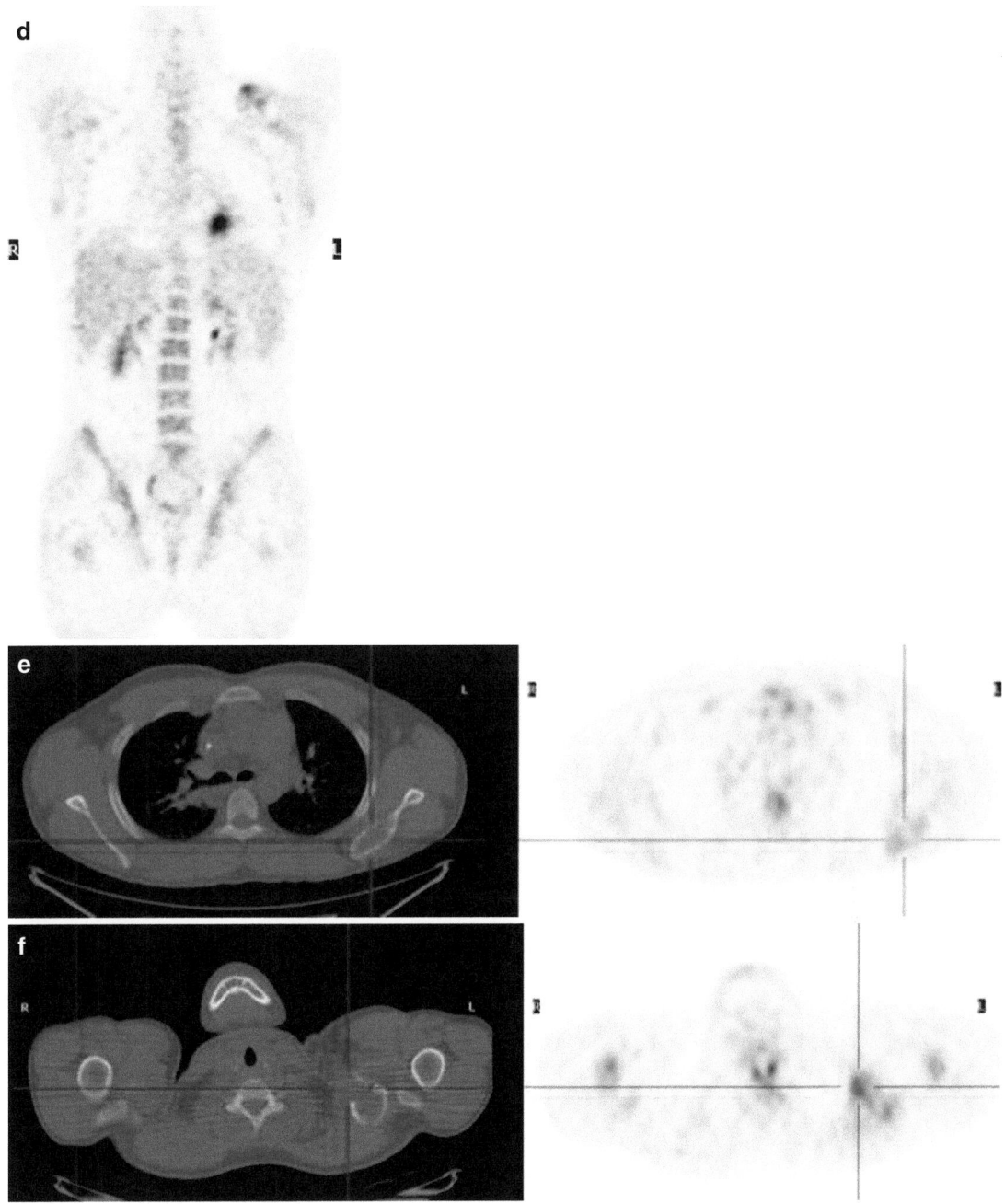

Fig. 6.6 (continued)

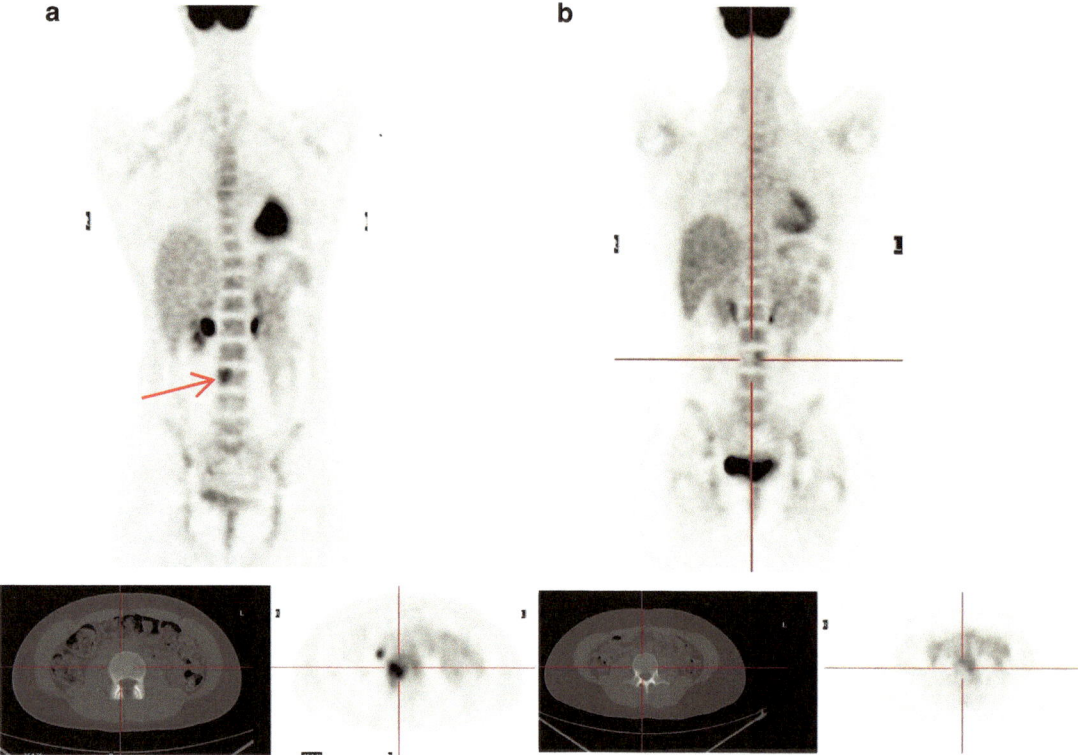

Fig. 6.7 Focal uptake in right side of L3 without abnormalities in CT due to bone marrow involvement at Baseline (*red arrow*: focal bone marrow uptake) (**a**); after treatment focal reduction of uptake due to bone marrow ablation (*mirror effect*) (**b**)

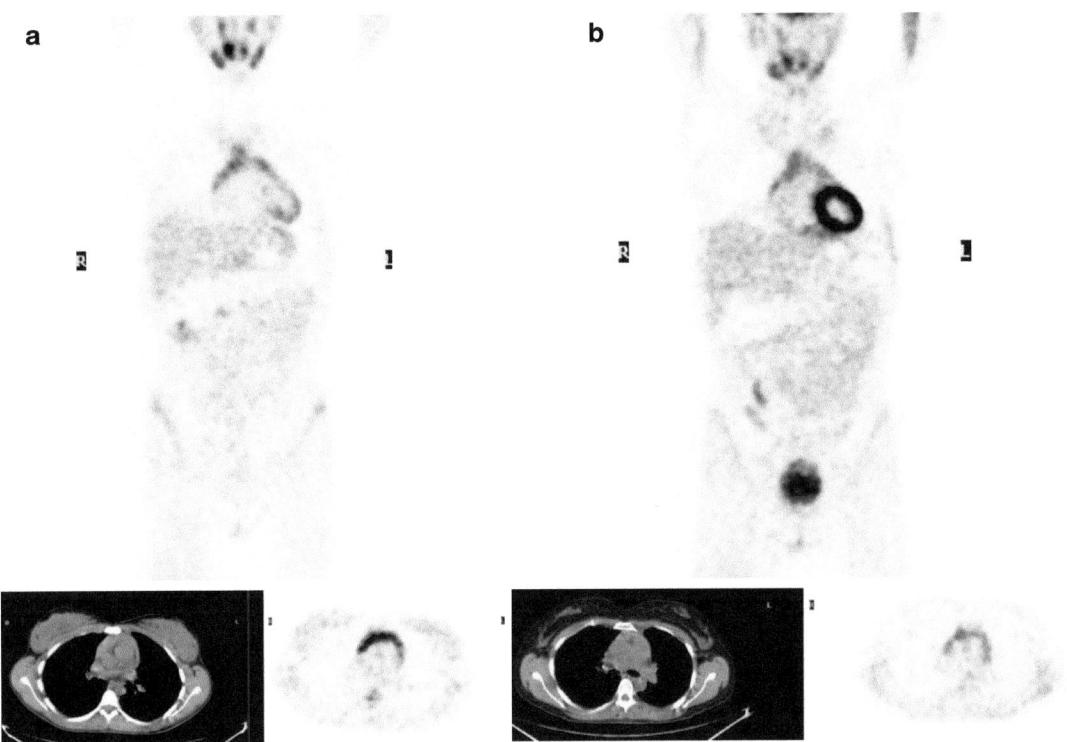

Fig. 6.8 Diffuse uptake in the anterior mediastinum due to thymic iperplasia 6 months (**a**) and 10 months (**b**) after the end of treatment for HL

| Baseline | Interim | End of therapy |

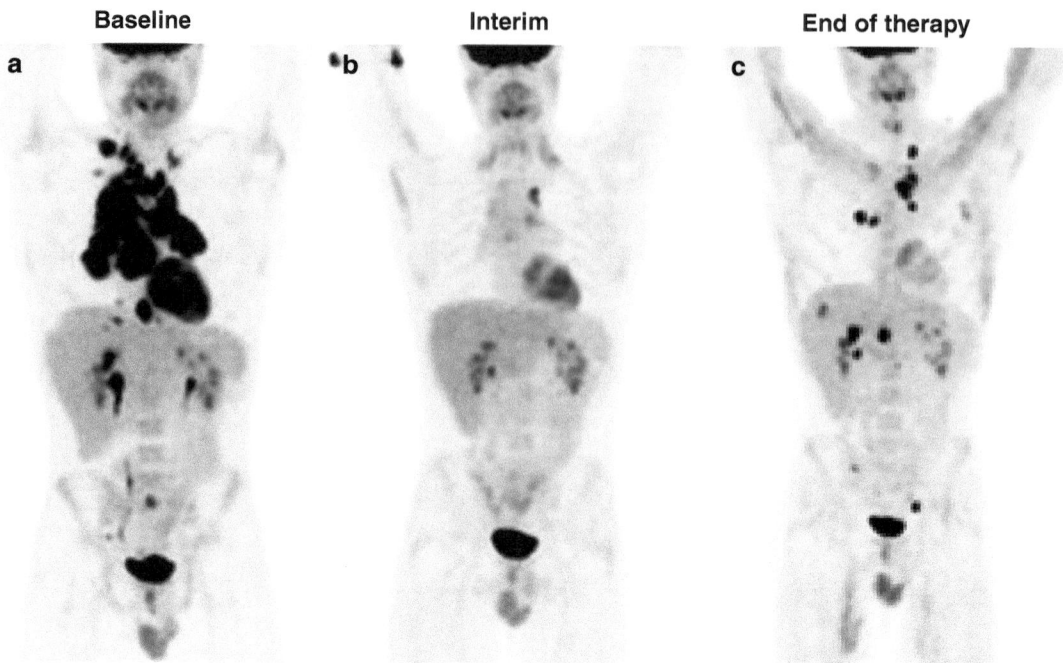

Fig. 6.9 (**a**) Stage IV HL; (**b**) PMR (score 4 upper mediastinal node) after 2 ABVD; (**c**) PMD at end of therapy after BEACOPP (new liver and bone lesion)

| Baseline | Interim | end of therapy |

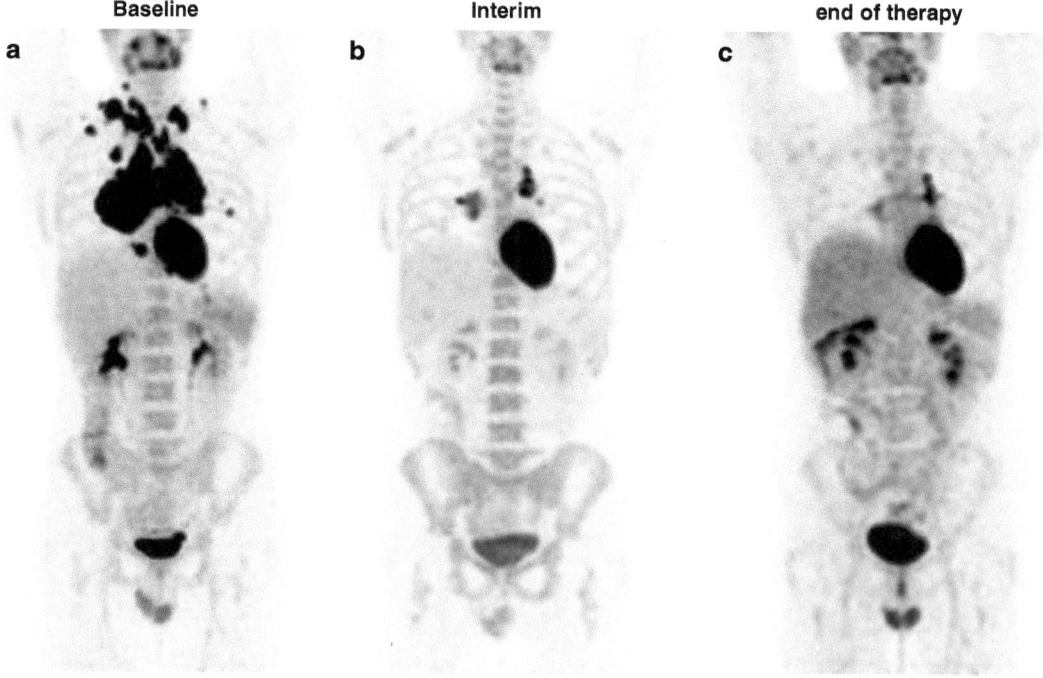

Fig. 6.10 (**a**) Stage IV HL (lung) HL; (**b**) residual disease in the pulmonary hilum (Score 4) (PMR); (**c**) Residual disease in the left pulmonary hilum after BEACOPP (Score 4) (PMR)

Site	Percentage
Nodal	
Cervical	55.8 (L); 47.4 (R)
Axillary	28.8 (L); 28.0 (R)
Infraclavicular	6.4 (L); 4.2 (R)
Hilar	23.0
Mediastinal	38.8
Periaortic	37.8
Pelvic	31.4 (L); 31.6 (R)
Inguinal	33.6 (L); 28.6 (R)
Extranodal	
Spleen	17.8
Bone marrow or bone	20.0
Lung	5.4
Liver	10.0
Bowel or gastric	5.4
Other nodal sites*	8.0

*Muscle, subcutaneous tissue, breast, and uterus.

Fig. 6.11 Example of template for reporting nodal and extranodal sites. In parenthesis the percentage of patients with lymphomatous involvement at specific nodal and extranodal sites [32]

References

1. Linee Guida per la Dematerializzazione della Documentazione Clinica in Diagnostica per Immagini, 4/4/2012, Conferenza permanente per i rapporti tra lo Stato, le Regioni e le provincie autonome di Trento e di Bolzano. www.statoregioni.it/dettaglio Doc.asp?idprov=10549&iddoc.
2. Boellard R, O'Doherty MJ, Weber WA, et al. FDG PET and PET/CT: EANM procedure guidelines for tumour PET imaging: version 1.0. Eur J Nucl Med Mol Imaging. 2010;37(1):181–200. doi:10.1007/s00259-009-1297-4.
3. Delbeke D, Coleman RE, Guiberteau MJ, et al. Procedure guidelines for tumour PET imaging with 18F-FDG PET/CT 1.0*. J Nucl Med. 2006;47:885–95.
4. Giordano A, Fanti S. Raccomandazioni Procedurali AIMN – Imaging Oncologico con 18F-FDG/PET – Vrs. 03/2012. www.aimn.it/pubblicazioni/LG/RP_AIMN_18F-oncologia.pdf.
5. 5th International workshop on PET in lymphoma. Palais de l'Europe. Menton, 19–20 Sept 2014. Organizing Committee M. Meignan, A. Gallamini, C. Haioun, S. Barrington, E. Itti, S. Luminari, E. Zucca. www.lymphomapet.com.
6. Barrington SF, Mikhaeel NG, Kostakoglu L, et al. Role of imaging in the staging and response assessment of lymphoma: consensus of the international conference on Malignant Lymphomas Imaging Working Group. doi:10.1200/JCO.2013.53.5229.
7. Cheson BD, Fisher RI, Barrington SF, et al. Recommendations for initial evaluation, staging, and response assessment of Hodgkin and non-Hodgkin lymphoma: the Lugano classification. doi:10.1200/JCO.2013.54.8800.
8. Cheson BD, Pfstner B, Juweid ME, et al. Revised response criteria for malignant lymphoma. J Clin Oncol. 2007;25:579–86.
9. Biggi A, Guerra L, Hofman MS. Current status of FDG-PET/CT in staging of adults lymphoma. Clin Transl Imaging. 2015. doi:10.1007/s40336-015-0127-x.
10. Rosemberg SA, Dorfman RF, Kaplan HS. The value of sequential bone marrow biopsy and laparotomy and splenectomy in a series of 127 consecutive untreated patients. Br J Cancer Suppl. 1975;2:221–7.
11. Khan AB, Barrington S, Mikhaeel NG, et al. PET-CT staging of DLBCL accurately identifies and provides new insight into the clinical significance of bone marrow involvement. Blood. 2013;122:61–7. doi:10.1182/blood2012-12-473389.
12. Adams HJA, Kwee TC, Fijnheer R, et al. Bone marrow 18-F-fluoro-2-deoxy-Dglucose positron emission tomography/computed tomography cannot replace bone marrow biopsy in diffuse large B-cell lymphoma. Am J Hematol. 2014;89:726–31.
13. Adams HJ, de Klerk JM, Fijnheer R, et al. Bone marrow biopsy in diffuse large B-cell lymphoma: useful or redundant test? Acta Oncol. 2015;54(1):67–72. doi:10.3109/0284186X.2014.958531.
14. Le Dortz L, De Guibert S, Bayat S, et al. Diagnostic and prognostic impact of 18F-FDG PET/CT in follicular lymphoma. Eur J Nucl Med Mol Imaging. 2010;37(12):2307–14. doi:10.1007/s00259-010-1539-5.
15. Wohrer S, Jaeger U, Kletter K, et al. 18F-fluorodeoxyglucose positron emission tomography (18F-FDG-PET) visualizes follicular lymphoma irrespective of grading. Ann Oncol Off J Eur Soc Med Oncol ESMO. 2006;17(5):780–4. doi:10.1093/annonc/mdl014.
16. Biggi A, Gallamini A, Chauvie S, et al. International validation study for interim PET in ABVD-treated, advanced-stage Hodgkin lymphoma: interpretation criteria and concordance rate among reviewers. J Nucl Med. 2013;54:683–90. doi:10.2967/jnumed.112.110890.
17. Bhargava P, Zhuang H, Kumar R, et al. Iatrogenic artifacts on whole-body F-18 FDG PET imaging. Clin Nucl Med. 2004;29(7):429–39.
18. Ulaner G, Lyall A. Identifying and distinguishing treatment effects and complications from malignancy at FDG PET/CT. Radiographics. 2013;33:1817–34.
19. Sarji A. Physiological uptake in FDG PET simulating disease. doi:10.2349/biij.2.4.e59. Available on line http://www.biij.org/2006/4/e59.
20. Mohei M, Abouzied MD, Elpida S, et al. 18F-FDG imaging: pitfalls and artifacts. J Nucl Med Technol. 2005;33:145–55.
21. Gontier E, Fourme E, Wartski M, et al. High and typical 18F-FDG bowel uptake in patients treated with metformin. Eur J Nucl Med Mol Imaging. 2008;35:95–9.
22. Oh JR, Song HC, Chong A, Ha JM, Jeong SY, Min JJ, Bom HS. Impact of medication discontinuation on increased intestinal FDG accumulation in diabetic patients treated with metformin. AJR Am J Roentgenol. 2010;195:1404–10.

23. Sugawara Y, Fisher SJ, Zasadny KR, et al. Preclinical and clinical studies of bone marrow uptake of fluorine-1-fluorodeoxyglucose with or without granulocyte colony-stimulating factor during chemotherapy. J Clin Oncol. 1998;16(1):173–80.

24. Sugawara Y, Zasadny KR, Kison PV, et al. Splenic fluorodeoxyglucose uptake increased by granulocyte colony-stimulating factor therapy: PET imaging results. J Nucl Med. 1999;40(9):1456–62.

25. Jerushalmi J, Frenkel A, Bar-Shalom R, et al. Physiologic thymic uptake of 18F-FDG in children and young adults: a PET/CT evaluation of incidence, patterns, and relationship to treatment. J Nucl Med. 2009;50(6):849–53.

26. Goethals I, Hoste P, De Vriendt C, et al. Time-dependent changes in 18F-FDG activity in the thymus and bone marrow following combination chemotherapy in paediatric patients with lymphoma. Eur J Nucl Med Mol Imaging. 2010;37(3):462–7.

27. Kirsch J, Arrossi AV, Yoon JK, et al. FDG positron emission tomography/computerized tomography features of bleomycin-induced pneumonitis. J Thorac Imaging. 2006;21(3):228–30.

28. Buchler T, Bomanji J, Lee SM. FDG-PET in bleomycin-induced pneumonitis following ABVD chemotherapy for Hodgkin's disease: a useful tool for monitoring pulmonary toxicity and disease activity. Haematologica. 2007;92(11):e120–1.

29. de Prost N, Tucci MR, Melo MF. Assessment of lung inflammation with 18F-FDG PET during acute lung injury. AJR Am J Roentgenol. 2010;195(2):292–300.

30. Faria S, Lisbona R, Stem J, et al. Is post-treatment FDG-PET/CT useful in differentiating tumor from fibrosis after curative radiation therapy (RT) alone for lung cancer? Int J Radiat Oncol Biol Phys. 2007;69(3 Suppl):S519–20.

31. Guerrero T, Johnson V, Hart J, et al. Radiation pneumonitis: local dose versus [18F]-fluorodeoxyglucose uptake response in irradiated lung. Int J Radiat Oncol Biol Phys. 2007;68(4):1030–5.

32. Hofman MS, Smeeton NC, Rankin SC, et al. Observer variation in interpreting 18F-FDG PET/CT findings for lymphoma staging. J Nucl Med. 2009;50:1594–7.

Index